1500pays
A Health Insurance Guide

Rochelle Wyatt

Ashley Demay

ISBN:1535202211
ISBN-13:9781535202213

DEDICATION

First of all, we dedicate this book to our family. We thank you for loving and supporting us in all that we do; unconditionally, daily and without fail. We don't have to name you by name because you already know who you are.

Secondly, we dedicate this book to our haters; the people that questioned our sanity, our wisdom, our timing and even our dreams. We don't have to name you by name because you already know who you are.

CONTENTS

ACKNOWLEDGMENTS

As a thank you from the 1500pays team for purchasing this book, we have added exclusive content not yet available on our website. Within these pages, we have included ten chapter tests; each with an answer key. A total of twenty case studies have been provided for you to try your hand at solving. In addition to this, you will gain access to three additional articles in chapter three, one additional article in chapter six, eight additional articles in chapter seven, as well as two additional chapters; eight and nine. We thank you for your purchase.

Please visit www.1500pays.com for more extras.

DISCLAIMER

The health insurance industry is not one-size-fits-all. This guide is an excellent source for the concise, in a nutshell, type of information you need when billing professional services. When in doubt, always defer to the health carrier for clarification and direction. Some parts of this book may reflect our personal opinions, observations and experiences. Please use this guide as yet another source of information.

1500PAYS A HEALTH INSURANCE GUIDE

This guide is for anyone in the medical billing arena with a simple wish - to obtain a better understanding of health insurance processes, plans and procedures. ***Anyone can put codes on a claim and hit the submit button. The test is in knowing how to take that claim and turn it into cash.***

The 1500pays Health Insurance Guide

Provides you with the information you need to take your knowledge of medical billing and coding to the next level. Maybe...

- ✓ You are a doctor and you need a little help with revenue management.
- ✓ You are a medical biller/receptionist/front office/back office assistant trying to gain a better understanding of the processes.
- ✓ You are a student taking medical billing and coding courses and need help studying.
- ✓ You are a new mom wanting to open a home based medical billing business one day.
- ✓ You've just completed a medical billing course but you lack the insurance expertise that is needed to secure your first job.
- ✓ You have a dispute with your insurance carrier about your own personal health claim and need help resolving the issue.

- ✓ You have an interest in medical billing and coding but have no idea where to start.

In 30 plus years, I have been exposed to just about all aspects of health insurance claim processing. I have billed claims to health insurance carriers, and on the reverse, I have worked for health insurance carriers by processing medical and dental claims. I have been a Medical Claim Auditor, a Preapproval, Reimbursement and Appeals Specialist and I have also worked in Provider Enrollment. I have worked with employers helping them to customize plans that fit their employee needs and I have spent time in Administration putting plan booklets and ID cards together. I am currently employed supervising the billing department of a large medical device company. After all of these years, what I know for sure is that medical billing is about setting expectations.

- What can I expect the patient to pay upfront?
- What am I expected to do, prior to the visit, to ensure accurate reimbursement?
- What am I expecting the health carrier to pay?
- Did the claim pay as expected?

This guide was designed to provide you with the overall health insurance knowledge that is needed to set your expectations and recover what is due.

Let me give you a real world example…

In my current position, occasionally we bring in temporary Medical Billers to assist with collections. Medical billing experience is required and health insurance knowledge is mandatory, however, I did agree to bring on a person who had just completed a medical billing course. Her task was to call health carriers to check the status on unpaid claims. She was asked to call the insurance carrier to check on a claim for $9000.00. Note: nothing was collected from the patient upfront. Here is how it went:

GREAT NEWS!!! INSURANCE PAID $2800
WHY SUCH A LOW PAYMENT?
THIS IS ALL THEY WOULD PAY
WHAT'S THE PLAN TYPE?
WAS IT THE RIGHT %AGE?
WHAT WERE WE EXPECTING?
? ? ? ? ?

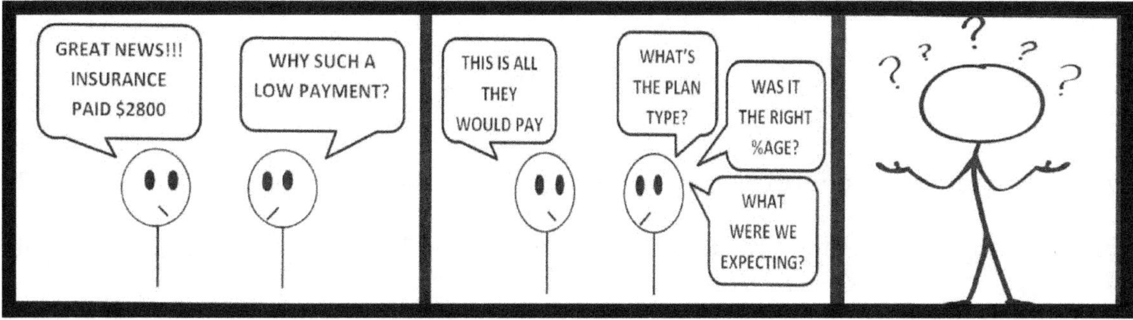

So without having a good understanding of health insurance, in general, how do you know the claim paid correctly?

Let's look at my expectations for this claim:

Patient has a PPO plan

80% in network - no deductible

50% out of network- $2000.00 deductible

$0 met at time of service.

Because we are an out of network provider, we had contacted the health plan, before the order was released, to negotiate for preapproval and a GAP exception. Both were granted. The patient had a secondary plan that we expected to pick up the eligible balance; hence, no payment was required from the patient up front.

We expected 100% of the allowed amount between the two carriers – with a small portion as write off. Clearly $2,800.00 paid on a $9,000.00 claim did not meet our expectations. We called the health carrier back to dispute this payment.

End of Story:

We were told by the health carrier that the claim had been paid out-of-network in error. In spite of the clean claim, the preapproval and the GAP exception - the claim was still paid incorrectly. Because we challenged the payment, the claim was ultimately paid as expected, by both carriers, with a small portion going to write off.

Please note: At ***no*** time during our calls to the health carrier did they "catch" the processing error that they made. Had we not bothered to pursue this issue, timely, we would have been stuck with a payment way less than expected.

The goal of this guide is to supplement what you already know about medical billing with the insurance knowledge that is needed to:

- ✓ Know that a claim has been coded correctly.
- ✓ Know how to bill a clean claim.
- ✓ Recover every dime that is due.

This field of medical billing is awesome, it is challenging, ever-changing and so necessary. Our hope is that this guide will provide you with the tools you need to do yourself proud.

Best wishes for a successful career,

The 1500pays Team

INSURANCE GUIDE

1 INSURANCE BASICS

Chapter Overview – Just like homeowners, life and auto, health insurance provides some protection against the high cost of health care. In this chapter, we provide a basic look at health insurance.

This Chapter Includes:

Affordable Care Act

Group Plans

Individual Plans

Universal Healthcare

Self-Funded

Employee Retirement Income Security Act

Fully Insured

Third Party Administrator

Health Insurance Portability and Accountability Act

AFFORDABLE CARE ACT

The Affordable Care Act (Obamacare) is a law that was passed with the goal of ensuring that the millions of Americans without health insurance would have access to healthcare.

When: It was signed into law on March 3, 2010 and required that every American have health insurance by March 31, 2014 or they would incur a tax penalty.

Why: The main purpose was to reduce the cost that the government pays toward healthcare. Both Medicare and Medicaid are government health plans.

How: The Affordable Care Act was signed into law in 2010 but was phased in over a 4-year period. See the key changes that were incurred each year.

Key changes in 2010

- Indoor tanning services were assessed a tax.
- Children were allowed to stay on their parent's plan until they turned 26.
- Private plans were required to cover preventive services with no co-payment, coinsurance or deductible.

- Insurance companies could not drop you from coverage for a serious condition.
- Insurance companies could not impose a lifetime coverage limit nor could they deny coverage to children with pre-existing conditions.

Key changes in 2011

- Medicare plans must offer preventive services with no deductibles or co-pay.
- Insurance companies must prove that they spent at least 80% of the premium payments on medical services, not other things like advertising or salaries.
- Health insurance companies have to submit justification for all rate hikes.

Key changes in 2012

- Health plans must begin to move away from paper records and must start to implement a more secure, confidential, electronic exchange of health information.

Key changes in 2013

- Manufacturers and importers of medical devices must pay a tax.
- Federal funds were increased so that Medicaid could offer no-cost preventive services.

Key changes in 2014

- Medicaid eligibility was expanded to include those with incomes up to 133% of the federal poverty level.
- Americans that do not purchase health insurance will be taxed.
- Insurance companies were prohibited from refusing to sell coverage or renew policies because of a pre-existing condition.

In a nutshell

The goal of the Affordable Care Act is to provide access to quality healthcare for all. Some people are under the impression that this really means free health insurance coverage for all. But for a large percentage of Americans, no cost health insurance coverage is just not an option.

To ease the burden placed by the uninsured, the Affordable Care Act did expand Medicaid coverage so that more people would qualify. It also provided cost incentives to those eligible citizens who were unable to qualify for Medicaid coverage but had difficulty paying premium costs.

In spite of its intent, the Affordable Care Act does not fully support the needs of all; including adults with lower incomes, the uninsured and the working poor. We still have many who may be insured yet they still are unable to afford the high out of pocket costs. Add to this, increased taxation, rising healthcare costs and poor reimbursement and you begin to understand why many people have called for the Affordable Care Act to be repealed.

So should the Affordable Care Act be repealed?

There has been a lot of opposition to the Affordable Care Act. Numerous lawsuits have been filed citing that it is unconstitutional to require people to buy healthcare insurance from a private carrier or pay a penalty. The Supreme Court ruled it was unconstitutional to impose a tax and the House of Representatives has voted to repeal the law numerous times.

Health insurance carriers have the burden of providing coverage to hundreds of new plan members; some of them with very serious health conditions. They continue to express concern over the ability to stay afloat in this climate of change.

To understand the issues with the Affordable Care Act, you have to understand how health insurance has always been structured.

- Health insurance coverage was usually voluntary, not mandatory.
- Typically, the young and healthy was the preferred plan member and the very sick were deemed to be uninsurable; or if insurable, the cost was very high.
- A health carrier could underwrite a plan to exclude or severely limit coverage for certain medical or preexisting conditions. For example, underwriting could refuse to cover any treatment related to a patient's high blood pressure for a pre-determined period of time or for the life of the plan.
- A carrier could drop you from coverage for a serious condition.
- Your premiums could be raised as deemed necessary by the health carrier.
- Employers could refuse to offer health insurance to their employees.
- Caring for the uninsured was shifted to the government or to private citizens in the form of higher health care costs and higher taxes.

The Affordable Care Act Changed Some of This By:

- Eliminating most preexisting limits, as long as you do not go more than 63 days without health coverage.
- Decreasing the uninsured by setting additional taxes for those that do not have health insurance. This is now tied into the filing of yearly tax returns.
- Eliminating the ability to be dropped due to a serious condition (as long the premium is paid).
- Requiring that health carriers seek "permission" to raise insurance rates.
- Establishing penalties for employers if they refuse to offer health insurance (for employers with over 50 full-time employees).
- Requiring that plans cover children to age 26.
- It has also expanded coverage for well care or preventative services with no upfront costs.

The Affordable Care Act changed all of this and more. Depending on what side you are on in this issue, clearly, it has its pluses and minuses.

Does the Affordable Care Act compare to Universal Care?

No. Universal Healthcare and the Affordable Care Act are not the same. Equal access to care with limited out of pocket costs expected under Universal Care is not represented under the Affordable Care Act.

Please note: My personal observations and opinions are represented in portions of this article. Do your homework to determine where you stand on this issue.

GROUP PLANS

Group health insurance plans are offered through your, or a family member's, place of employment and allows for a number of people to be covered by a single policy that is issued to their employer.

Employers that decide to provide health insurance to their employees may contact an Insurance Agent or Broker to do the legwork or they can contact an insurance carrier directly. Most insurance companies offer a wide range of coverage options that can be tailor-made to fit each employer's "wish list" of desired coverages.

Employers can customize the plan to be anything from a traditional fee-for-service plan to one of the many managed care plans. Incidental coverages like dental, vision and prescription drug coverage are also available. The final benefits that are ultimately offered to employees are usually made up of a mixture of some or all of the following:

- The carrier's suggested benefits.
- The standard coverages.
- The state mandated coverages.
- The employer's list of "must haves."
- The employee's list of "must haves."
- The financial needs of the company.

Healthcare coverage is expensive and employers may choose to omit a desired benefit simply because it may be cost prohibitive to the plan.

Before accepting a group, the insurance carrier will evaluate the entire group of employees as a whole; looking at ages, sex, health, occupation, avocation, lifestyle and past claims history to determine if a group is an acceptable risk. Once a group is accepted, the final benefit, coverage, premium, and eligibility issues are ironed out and the master policy is issued as a contract between the employer and the insurance company. Members of the plan are not a party to this contract.

In lieu of copies of the Master policy, members of the plan are provided with a Certificate of Coverage or a Benefit Booklet that outlines the benefits under the plan. Members of the plan will also be issued ID Cards that provide the member's name, identification, member and/or group numbers as well as the insurance carrier's telephone numbers and addresses.

Employers can choose to provide healthcare at no cost to the employees by paying the full premium or they can require that employees contribute toward the cost of healthcare by paying a portion of the premium.

New hires become eligible under the health plan after completion of the plan's waiting period, which could happen immediately, the first of the next month, 90 days or even beyond.

Employers usually offer a period, once per year, for employees to drop, add or make changes to their existing health coverage. This period is referred to as open enrollment.

The employer is responsible for paying the full premium to the insurance carrier, usually on a monthly basis. Upon receipt of the premium, the insurance carrier will credit the employer's account and keep each employee's coverage active. Failure to receive the required premium may result in withholding of claim payments and/or termination of group coverage. Since this is a group plan, the actions of one affect the group as a whole. This means if only a portion of the premium is paid, the entire group will be lapsed.

The employer is also responsible for advising the insurance carrier of any new hires and/or situations where an employee may no longer qualify for coverage such as terminations, reduction in hours, COBRA members, or any other change that may affect eligibility.

The insurance company is usually responsible for maintaining correct eligibility and enrollment information, providing ID cards and plan booklets, providing customer support and processing all claims in accordance with the provisions of the plan.

Every year, active groups will go through a renewal process. During this time, the insurance carrier will look at the group's overall claim history, experience, etc., to determine if a premium increase is warranted.

A large amount of claim activity, for example, a seriously ill employee or a pre term baby, could result in higher than average claim payments being made by the carrier. The carrier may pass this increase on to the employer in the form of a premium increase. The employer may choose to pass this increase on to his employees by increasing the amount that they contribute toward health insurance.

Although the insurance carrier may feel that a rate increase is warranted, the employer has the final option to either accept the premium increase as stated or they can shop for insurance coverage elsewhere.

Normally, employees feel that they have no choice but to accept the benefits that are provided by an employer and to accept the insurance carrier's handling of a claim. Very often, a plan fails to provide adequate benefits and/or an insurance carrier fails to provide good service, timely processing and adequate reimbursement of claims.

Employees should always advise their Employer/Human Resources Department about inadequate benefits and poor service by the insurance company. Employers may decide to restructure the benefits or switch insurance carriers based on this feedback.

Claim disputes do arise and most can be settled by contacting the insurance carrier to appeal the handling of a claim. If the health carrier is unable or unwilling to resolve an issue to your satisfaction, you have the option of asking the patient to take this one step further.

- For fully-insured plans: The plan member can file a complaint with the Department of Insurance (DOI) for their particular state. The DOI will work with the member and the insurance carrier to get an issue resolved.
- For self-funded plans: The plan member can contact the Department of Labor who will work with them to try to get an issue resolved.

INDIVIDUAL PLANS

An individual health insurance plan is an option for those whose employer does not offer health insurance coverage or for those who are self-employed, unemployed or have a serious health condition. Individual plans provide coverage for the individual and their dependents only.

Most insurance companies offer a nice range of coverage options for individual plans; from the traditional fee-for-service plans to one of the numerous types of managed care plans. Incidental coverages like dental, vision and prescription drug are also available.

The final benefits are usually made up of a mixture of some or all of the following:

- The applicant's list of "must haves."
- The carrier's suggested benefits.
- The standard benefits.
- The state mandated benefits.
- What the applicant can afford.

Before an individual policy is issued, the insurance carrier will evaluate the applicant and dependents to determine if they are an acceptable risk. Once accepted, the final benefit, coverage, premium and eligibility issues are ironed out and the policy is issued as a contract between the applicant(s) and the insurance company.

Members of the plan will also be issued ID cards that provide the member's name, identification, member, and/or group numbers as well as the insurance carrier's telephone numbers and addresses.

Unlike a group plan where you can expect lower premiums because you have several members to share in the cost of health insurance, the cost for an individual plan is usually much more expensive. Due to more stringent underwriting guidelines, individual plans can be more difficult to obtain at affordable prices; especially for those with chronic, serious or any medical condition with the potential to incur large costs.

The member is responsible for paying all premiums to the insurance carrier, usually on a monthly basis. Upon receipt of the premium, the insurance carrier will credit the member's account and keep the coverage active. Failure to receive the required premium may result in withholding of claim payments or termination of coverage.

The insurance company is responsible for maintaining correct eligibility, providing customer support and processing all claims in accordance with the provisions of the plan. Remember the plan is written and agreed to, by contract, between the insurance carrier and the member.

Every year, members with individual coverage may go through a renewal process. During this time, the insurance carrier will look at the overall claim history, experience, etc., to determine if a premium increase is warranted.

A large amount of claim activity could result in higher than average claim payments being made by the carrier. The carrier may pass this increase on to the member in the form of a premium increase. Although the insurance carrier may feel that a rate increase is warranted, the member has the final option to either dispute or accept the premium increase or they can shop for insurance coverage elsewhere.

Because of the difficulties in obtaining health coverage, members of individual plans have more of a tendency to stay with a current plan, even if the plan fails to provide adequate benefits, the premiums are high, and/or the insurance carrier fails to provide good service, timely processing and adequate reimbursement of claims.

Members of individual plans should not simply accept poor service. These types of claim issues do arise and most can be settled by contacting the insurance carrier to appeal or complain about the way you or your claim was handled.

Unresolved claim disputes or problems can be directed to the Department of Insurance (DOI) for that state. The DOI will work with you and the insurance carrier to get your issues resolved.

UNIVERSAL HEALTHCARE

Universal healthcare is designed to provide all citizens of a particular country equal access to quality healthcare. Its goal is to ensure that no one will be without health coverage should they need it nor will they have to worry about incurring huge out of pocket costs.

The way that healthcare is delivered can be complex and economically driven, leaving the most needy with limited access to the medical care that they need, simply because they cannot afford it. This translates into health care costs for the uninsured that must be absorbed somewhere; increased burden on the insured, higher taxes, out of control health care costs or a combination of the three.

Universal Healthcare was designed to bridge that gap by finding ways to fund healthcare coverage for all citizens of that particular country.

Citizens and/or other entities may be responsible for paying all health care premiums. These entities, like the government for one, has a vested interest in prompting wellness and healthy living. The connection between good medical and preventative care and lower health care costs is evident. Some countries like Canada, for one, have adopted some very strict health regulations and have banned some of the "unhealthy" foods and drinks that are common in America.

Universal Healthcare has numerous different funding systems, from employers to private citizens to the government. Countries that offer Universal Healthcare, are also encouraged to find alternative ways to fund healthcare for all of its citizens; perhaps by adding special taxes for some goods like tobacco and alcohol or by having community based health plans. Private health plans may also be available as a supplement to their current coverage.

Universal Healthcare is not a perfect solution and it is not without some negatives. Not all services are covered for everyone and exclusions for certain conditions and treatments could apply. Some patients have even been required to go on waiting lists for certain treatments and services resulting in a delay of months and even years for medical care and even surgery. Some frustrated with the level of care under Universal healthcare have migrated to America to have health care services performed.

Universal Healthcare costs are paid for in various ways, including:

- **Single Payer -** Health care is paid by the government.
- **Tax-Based Financing -** Individuals are assessed taxes.
- **Social Health Insurance -** Costs are paid by workers, the self-employed, businesses and/or government.
- **Community-Based Health Insurance -** Members of a specific community all make payments to a health fund that they use when they need medical care.

How does the Affordable Care Act compare to Universal Care?

Universal Healthcare and the Affordable Care Act are not the same. The expectation of equal access to care with low out of pocket costs under Universal Care is not represented under the Affordable Care Act.

The Affordable Care Act (Obamacare) is but one of the many healthcare delivery options in America. The other options being Medicare, Medicaid, employer group plans, individual plans, etc., all have a wide range of plan designs, benefits, provisions and provider access. But despite the vast array of options, America still has a large number of citizens without any form of health insurance coverage, and others who, although insured, are unable to afford the huge out of pocket costs.

The following lists the countries who have some form of Universal Care:

Norway, New Zealand, Japan, Germany, Belgium, United Kingdom, Kuwait, Sweden, Bahrain, Brunei, Canada, Netherlands, Austria, United Arab Emirates, Finland, Slovenia, Denmark, Luxembourg, France, Australia, Ireland, Italy, Portugal, Cyprus, Greece, Spain, South Korea, Iceland, Hong Kong, Singapore, Switzerland, Israel.

SELF-FUNDED

A self-funded plan, also called a self-insured plan, works the same as a fully insured plan except that for self-funded plans the financial responsibility for paying all healthcare claims will be bore, either partially or fully, by the employer instead of the insurance carrier.

An employer may choose to self-fund a plan to:

- Have more visibility into the overall health of the plan. This can help to minimize costs by identifying plan members and/or dependents that are seriously ill or injured in order to manage costs early on.
- Serve as the final decision maker for any service or treatment that may be outside of the current plan design.
- Extend the funds needed to pay all claims but also have the ability to keep any unused premium dollars that are held on account, earning interest, should claim payments be less than expected.

The employer must have the funds to pay all claims incurred by the group of employees. This concept can be risky because the employer's finances could take a huge hit if a catastrophic claim or more claims than expected are presented for payment. Claim volume could change every month making it difficult to predict what could be paid out. To limit the potential loss, an employer could purchase Stop Loss and/or

Reinsurance Coverage. Stop Loss coverage reimburses the employer if a ***particular*** claim goes over a certain dollar amount and Reinsurance Coverage reimburses the employer when ***all*** claims for the group go over a certain amount.

Since most employers do not have the facilities to process claims on site, they may enter into an arrangement with an organization to administer the policy as written. This organization will handle the customer service, collect premiums, issue ID cards, provide benefit and eligibility information and process claims. However, the employer is the final decision maker. This arrangement is called Administrative Services Only (ASO) and this type of arrangement is usually handled by a Third Party Administrator (TPA). The employer is responsible for paying the costs to administer the plan.

So why is it important to know who is at risk for claims?

In most cases, the fact that a plan is fully insured or self-funded is invisible to plan members and does not matter at all, unless of course when something is not processed as expected. The appeal process is where you will need to know if you are dealing with a fully insured or self-funded plan. Self-funded plans are regulated by ERISA, the Employee Retirement Income Security Act. ERISA plans require uniformity. This means that the employer has a special responsibility to protect all covered employee's interests.

ERISA plans fall under the protection of the US Department of Labor. The Department of Insurance, for that particular state, will be unable to assist with complaints from members that are covered under a self-funded plan. For claims that were not paid as expected and an appeal is needed, you would need to:

- Check the Summary Plan Description (SPD) to see if the benefits are included in your plan.
- Appeal to the Health Plan Administrator or your Employer.

If not satisfied with the decision, you can appeal to the US Department of Labor.

EMPLOYEE RETIREMENT INCOME SECURITY ACT

ERISA is one of the many buzzwords that you hear about in the health insurance industry. ERISA applies to private (non-government) employers that offer employer-sponsored health insurance plans. ERISA does not apply to private plans or individual insurance policies.

ERISA – the Employee Retirement Income Security Act of 1974, sets the standard on how participants under pension and health plans must be protected. ERISA does not mandate that an employer provide health insurance to its employees; but, if offered, it regulates how the health plan must behave.

ERISA plans include some important protections:

- The Consolidated Omnibus Budget Reconciliation Act (COBRA) of 1985 allows employees and beneficiaries the right to continue coverage under the Employer's plan for a limited time after they lose employment.
- The Health Insurance Portability and Accountability Act (HIPAA) of 1996, limits a health plan from denying claims for a pre-existing medical condition as well as any other health based discrimination.
- Newborns' and Mothers' Health Protection Act states that a plan that offers maternity coverage has to pay for at least a 48-hour hospital stay following childbirth (96-hour stay in the case of a caesarean

section).

- Mental Health Parity Act requires that annual or lifetime limits for mental health benefits can be no lower than any other medical or surgical benefit.
- Women's Health and Cancer Rights Act protects patients who elect for breast reconstruction surgery in connection with a mastectomy.

In addition, ERISA...

- Regulates how a managed care plan must act.
- Requires reporting and accountability to the Federal Government.
- States that plan members must be given a Summary Plan Description that outlines the benefits and provisions of the plan.
- Requires written processes on how a claim should be filed and how to appeal if denied.

ERISA is important to employees, providers and billers?.

Many years ago when I first started out in the insurance industry, it was not uncommon for a me to spend a great amount of my time appealing for coverage for services that were denied by the health carrier for some reason or another. The first thing I would do is ask the patient for a copy of their Summary Plan Description (SPD). The SPD helped me to understand if I even had a basis for appeal.

ERISA requires that all plan members be provided with a Summary Plan Description. A Summary Plan Description is often referred to as a plan booklet and is provided to all plan members upon enrollment. It provides pages and pages of information on all aspects of the plan including:

- What is covered
- Available benefits

- Plan Limits
- How the plan operates
- When coverage starts
- When it ends
- Who is eligible for coverage
- Your rights when you are terminated
- What is not covered

Today, occasionally, I still refer to a patient's SPD to help me appeal a complex denial.

Real Word Example

Recently, I had a carrier deny a service based on the age of the patient. After referring to ALL pages of their SPD, I could not find anywhere that stated that the service in question was age specific. The appeal was presented to the carrier along with a copy of the appropriate section in the SPD. The denial was overturned and the approval was granted.

Of course, this goes the other way as well. Had this plan clearly stated the age requirement, I would have known that it was a waste of time to appeal to the carrier and the patient would have been advised of their options before proceeding with the service.

FULLY-INSURED

Fully insured means that the insurance carrier, not the employer, is responsible for paying all claims incurred by the group of employees. Employers that choose a fully insured plan do not want to assume the financial risk associated with health claims because the overall financial health of the company could take a huge hit if a catastrophic claim, or more claims than expected, are presented for payment. The employer would rather assign this risk over to the insurance carrier.

Employers that choose a fully insured plan will be rated by the insurance carrier who will assess the overall "risk" of the group including the number of employees, ages, health, etc. The health carrier will guesstimate what they perceive the potential costs could be for the group, trend this number up a bit and add in the cost to administer the plan as written in order to come up with a monthly premium that the employer will be required to pay to keep the coverage active. Failure to remit payment timely will result in a lapse in coverage for all members of the plan. No eligibility and no claims payments will be made until the account is brought current.

Employers may pay all of the premium costs or they may require the group of employees to contribute towards the cost as well. The goal is that the premiums collected will be enough to cover ALL claims that come in, as well as the costs to administer the plan. Any overage will be the insurance carrier's profit. On the reverse, the health carrier will be responsible for paying any shortage, either due to inadequate premium collection or higher than expected claim volume or costs.

Employers are usually locked into that premium rate for one year; unless more employees are added. After one year, the insurance carrier will review the claim history and overall health of the group to decide if a premium increase is warranted. At that time, the employer can accept the premium increase (it may be passed on to the employees who will see more money taken out of their checks for healthcare) or the employer can switch to another insurance carrier who will guarantee a lower rate.

So why does it matter if a plan is fully insured?

How the plan is administered is usually invisible to the plan members and really does not matter except in the case of appeals. If coverage is denied or a claim is not paid as expected, before the appeal is started, you will want to know if this plan is fully or self-insured. This gives a clear idea on how the appeal process should be handled.

To appeal a fully-insured claim:

1. Review the back of the EOB to determine the appeal process.
2. Normally, a call can be placed to the health carrier to try to get the issue resolved by phone.
3. If unable to resolve by phone, a written appeal will be sent to the health carrier who will determine if the claim was processed correctly based on the plan benefits.
4. Once all appeal options have been exhausted and you are still unsatisfied, the PATIENT can file a complaint with their state's Department of Insurance.

The Department of Insurance will work on the patient's behalf by contacting the health carrier to try to get the issue resolved.

THIRD PARTY ADMINISTRATOR

Third Party Administrator (TPA) is an independent company that is paid by the employer to handle the administrative tasks related to the health insurance plan.

Some employers may choose to self-fund the health insurance plan that they offer to their employees. This means that all health claims that are incurred by the group of employees and their dependents will be paid by the employer instead of the health insurance carrier.

Some of the benefits for the employer to self-fund include:

- It provides a detailed look at the overall health of the plan so that they can proactively try to manage the level of care to minimize costs.
- They will be the final decision maker for any services or treatment that may be outside the current plan design.
- They would be able to keep any unused premium dollars that are held on account, earning interest.

Claim processing and plan administration requires a great deal of skill, knowledge and expertise and most employers simply do not have the staff nor do they wish to spend the time and money needed to develop a team that can handle the claim function in-house. They would rather use a Third Party Administrator (TPA).

A Third Party Administrator allows the employer to outsource the claim administration and claim handling portion to an outside company that specializes in making this process invisible to the plan members. The Third Party Administrator could, based on the needs of the employer, handle all or part of the claim processing and plan administration responsibilities, including:

- Plan enrollments
- Issuing ID cards
- Collecting premiums
- Paying claims
- COBRA administration
- Reporting

The Third Party Administrator charges a fee for the services that they provide and that fee could be on a per claim, per employee, per service, incurred claims or any other basis as determined by the Third Party Administrator.

So why does this matter?

In truth, this really has no bearing at all on claim processing. The medical billing process is the same and the Third Party Administrator manages the claim handling process and plan administration just like a health insurance carrier would - in accordance with the plan provisions and benefits.

In most cases, the patient, the provider of service nor the medical biller will have any idea that a plan is fully insured by the insurance carrier or self-funded by the employer. The Third Party Administrator's goal is to make the process seamless to plan members.

HEALTH INSURANCE PORTABILITY AND ACCOUNTABILITY ACT

HIPAA, Health Insurance Portability and Accountability Act of 1996, is a federal law that was written to address a long list of health care related issues. In this guide, we will address two aspects of HIPAA, Title I and II. Title I provides protection for plan members when they switch from one group plan to another or lose their job. Title II calls for national standards of how healthcare data is transmitted and protected.

Title I

Title I addresses the requirements for how members covered under group, and some individual health, plans should be protected.

HIPAA states that:

- A health plan cannot deny you because of your health.
- Pre-existing condition waiting periods must be limited.
- For some employees and individuals, HIPAA guarantees the renewal and availability of health coverage.
- Pregnancy cannot be considered a pre-existing condition.
- You cannot be denied coverage for mental illness, a genetic flaw, a disability or because of your past

claims history.

One of the key features was that HIPAA allows you to get "credit" for the time you have been insured under a previous health plan and allows you to use this credit with your new health plan, as long as the coverage is considered credible.

Credible coverage means coverage under a government or church plan, group or individual health plan, Medicare, Medicaid and Champus, Indian Health Service, state high risk pools, or coverage for federal employees.

For example

You have worked for ABC Company for 3 years and you decide to go to work for XYZ Company. Provided that you have no lapse in coverage of more than 63 days, you cannot be subject to a pre-existing period. The new employer is required to honor any time that you were insured under a prior plan.

Title II

Title II addresses the standards for protection of a patient's health information, including privacy and security.

So what is Protected Health Information (PHI)?

PHI is:

- Any and all information that you have or have access to about a person's past, current or future medical conditions both physical and mental.
- Any information that can be used to identify or link any type of treatment, services or diagnosis to a particular person including their name, address, date of birth, social security number, ID number, etc.

By all, it means **ALL** health care providers that handle any aspect of the health insurance process themselves or that use an outside billing service. This requirement for the protection and security of all patient information applies to health insurance carriers, clearinghouses, and any and all healthcare providers that bill claims, verify benefits and eligibility, handle referrals and authorization requests, or any other healthcare related process or procedure. This includes all providers of healthcare services, including:

- Hospitals
- Physicians
- Dentists
- Clearinghouses when acting as a business associate to a provider of medical services.
- Any other person or organization that provides a medical service, bills claims and is reimbursed for healthcare services.

Severe penalties are in place for any provider of service or business associate that fails to keep a person's protected health information private and secure and who fails to notify when a breach of personal data has occurred.

What is a Business Associate?

Outside medical billing companies do not have direct access to patient's information. All claims information is passed from the provider to the billing company. However, medical billing companies that submit claims on a provider's behalf, are required to sign a Business Associate Agreement.

A Business Associate Agreement is a legal document signed by the provider and billing company ensuring that everyone is clear on how this shared data should be protected and kept secure. The provider is entrusting a patient's medical information to the billing company who, by signature, agrees to fully protect all patient data. With this agreement, the billing company understands the legal requirements for protected health information and is fully aware of the processes as well as the violations and requirements should any data be breached.

In a nutshell

Simply put, we are the keepers of Protected Health Information and we have a legal requirement and a personal obligation to keep **ALL** patients' health information safe and secure.

This means that only those with a ***need to know*** should have access to a patient's protected health information.

Wanting to know, interested in and being curious about does not meet the standard of need to know. If someone is not directly related to the billing process, then they should have ZERO access to a patient's health information.

CHAPTER ONE TEST

Directions: Using what you have learned in Chapter One, answer the following questions.

1. What is the purpose of the Affordable Care Act?

2. What is the difference between the Affordable Care Act and Universal Healthcare?

3. List two reasons why an employer would choose to self-fund a health insurance plan?

4. How does ERISA affect the health insurance process?

5. What is credible coverage?

6. If claim expenses exceed the total premium that was collected, who is responsible for paying the overage on a self-funded plan?

7. Would a fully insured plan need to use a TPA?

8. What does ASO stand for?

9. What is a Business Associate Agreement?

10. What is the difference between an individual plan and a group plan?

11. The media has hinted about a well know celebrity's current health crisis and you have access to their health records. Since everyone "knows" about it already, can you look at their file and disclose what you know? Explain.

2 PLAN TYPES

Chapter Overview – PPO or HMO? What is Medigap coverage? What are the advantages of one type of plan over another? We will answer those questions for you in this chapter as we take a detailed look into the most common plan types.

This Chapter Includes:

Preferred Provider Organization

Exclusive Provider Organization

Health Maintenance Organization

Point Of Service

Fee For Service

Commercial Plans

Medicaid

Medicare

Medigap

Military

Workers Compensation

Blue Cross Blue Shield

Managed Care Plans

PREFERRED PROVIDER ORGANIZATION

What is a PPO?

A Preferred Provider Organization (PPO) is offered by insurance companies and is a group, or network, of providers of all specialties who, in exchange for greater access to plan members, have agreed to provide healthcare at discounted fees, or contracted rates. The contracted rates are determined by the insurance company and are agreed to, by contract, between them and the provider. To ensure that providers are able to capture their share of patients, they usually will participate in numerous PPO networks.

As an incentive for patients to use PPO providers, they can expect no/low deductible and a higher level of reimbursement if in network providers are used. Services by out of network doctors are subject to a higher deductible and a lower level of reimbursement.

Participating providers agree not to bill the patient and write off any amounts over the contracted rate. However, they are allowed to collect any applicable deductible and co-insurance amounts required. Non-participating providers may have their claims adjudicated based on the Usual, Customary, or Reasonable (UCR) allowance, a percentage of the contracted rate or any other method as determined by the insurance company. They are allowed to collect any amount not paid by the insurance company.

EXAMPLE OF A PPO PLAN DESIGN

IN NETWORK:

PLAN PAYS 90%

PATIENT PAYS 10% OF COVERED CHARGES UP TO A MAX OF $1500.00

PLAN PAYS 100% AFTER $1500.00 IS PAID OUT OF POCKET.

OUT OF NETWORK:

$100.00 DEDUCTIBLE

PLAN PAYS 70%

PATIENT PAYS 30% OF COVERED CHARGES UP TO A MAX OF $3000.00

PLAN PAYS 100% AFTER $3000.00 IS PAID OUT OF POCKET.

Let's look at two examples on how a claim will be processed with in-network and out-of-network providers.

IN-NETWORK SCENARIO:

James goes to an in network doctor and with an office visit, lab and x-ray, he incurs $540.00 in medical expenses. The claim was billed to the health carrier and they allowed $440.00 of the claim.

So what did James have to pay out of his pocket for this visit?

PATIENT RESPONSIBILITY:

$440.00 x (10%) = $44.00

JAMES IS RESPONSIBLE FOR $44.00

HEALTH CARRIER RESPONSIBILITY:

$440.00 x (90%) = $396.00

HEALTH CARRIER WILL PAY $396.00

Provider was paid: $44.00 (patient) + $396.00 (carrier) = $440.00

Note: $100.00 over the contracted rate is adjusted off.

OUT-OF-NETWORK SCENARIO:

James goes to an out of network doctor and with an office visit, lab and x-ray, he incurs $550.00 in medical expenses. The claim was billed to the health carrier and they allowed $450.00 of the claim. Let's assume that none of the deductible was met.

So what did James have to pay out of his pocket for this visit?

PATIENT RESPONSIBLITY:

Billed $550 - $100 (Not Covered) = $450

$450 - $100 (Deductible) = $350

$350 x (30%) = $105.

Patient will pay $305
[$100 (Not Covered) + $100 (Deductible) + $105 ($350 x 30%)]

HEALTH CARRIER RESPONSIBILITY:

Billed $550 - $100 (Not Covered) = $450

$450 - $100 (Deductible) = $350

$350 x (70%) = $245

Health Carrier will pay $245

Provider was paid $305.00 (patient) + $245.00 (carrier) = $550.00

Note: The patient was responsible for the $100.00 not covered amount.

Don't assume that something in the way a claim is coded, identifies it as a claim that should be processed at the in network benefit level. There is no way to bill a claim as "in network" or "out of network." That part of the magic happens when the claim is processed by the health carrier. Don't assume that just because you are a participating provider that your claim will be paid correctly. Review all EOB's and dispute all incorrect payments.

ADVANTAGES & DISADVANTAGES OF PPO PLANS

Advantage to Members Participating in PPO Plans

- Members have the freedom to select any doctor, in network or out of network.
- They can see any doctor or specialist without having to wait for a referral.
- Members who use in network providers can expect higher reimbursement with low or no deductible.

Disadvantages to Members Participating in PPO Plans

- If out of network treatment is sought, the member can expect to pay higher out of pocket expenses.

Advantages to Providers Participating in PPO Plans

- Providers may be listed in the directories of several different networks, which may result in an increase in the number of new patients.

Disadvantage to Providers Participating in PPO Plans

- The reality is that doctors may be working harder, seeing more patients, because reimbursement based on contracted rates is normally lower than what the provider may bill for a same service and they cannot make the patient responsible for the difference.

PPO plans usually have some portion that a patient is required to pay upfront. Collect this at the time of service.

PPO plans have a wide range of coverages and benefits and no two plans may be alike; even plans written by the same carrier. Always check benefits and eligibility before services are rendered. If 30 days has passed since the patient was seen, check again.

EXCLUSIVE PROVIDER ORGANIZATION

An Exclusive Provider Organization (EPO) is a type of managed care plan that is offered by insurance companies. Exclusive is the word that best describes how this plan functions. Either use the limited list of participating providers or pay the full cost for treatment.

An Exclusive Provider Organization plan pays ZERO for out of network services.

The only exceptions to the zero out of network policy maybe for:

- Situations where emergency care is needed. The plan understands that no one will have the wherewithal to consult the plan directory to try to locate an in network provider in an emergency. But be prepared, once the patient stabilizes they will be moved to an in network hospital.
- When the plan does not have anyone in network that can provide the care that the patient needs. That care better be medically necessary and approved by the plan in advance.

An Exclusive Provider Organization plan is all about keeping healthcare costs as low as possible.

- Members are required to use only in network providers or pay for all services out of pocket.
- Pre-approval may be required for all mid to high dollar services and all specialty care.

- Providers are paid at a contacted rate or some other type of payment methodology as determined by the carrier.

On the reverse, the features that make an EPO attractive are:

- Patients normally pay little out of their pocket because the plan requires little in the form of patient costs; low or no copays, deductibles and coinsurance amounts.
- You do not have to have a primary care doctor to manage all aspects of your healthcare.
- No referrals are needed. You can see any provider you want in the network without waiting.
- The plan is cheaper. Lower premium costs means less is taken out of the plan member's paycheck.

I work with all kinds of health insurance plans nationwide and EPO plans are the plans that I work with the least. In spite of the low out of pocket costs, the exclusivity of the plan may be the reason why.

In my opinion, what ranks highest when choosing a health plan is making sure that the health providers you visit often are part of the network. Most people are just not willing to give up that great pediatrician that their kids love or the family doctor that they can count on just to save a few dollars.

Because an EPO is so exclusive, it limits access to a huge list of providers that one would expect to see under a larger managed care plan.

ADVANTAGES & DISADVANTAGES OF EPO PLANS

Advantages to Members Participating in EPO Plans

- Less out of pocket expense due to the higher reimbursement for in network providers.

Disadvantages to Members Participating in EPO Plans

- Small network of providers to choose from.
- Charges for out of network providers will not be reimbursed.

Advantages to Providers Participating in EPO Plans

- Less doctors to compete for patients.

Disadvantages to Providers Participating in EPO Plans

- Increase in patients, may not justify the lower reimbursement.

HEALTH MAINTENANCE ORGANIZATION

Health Maintenance Organizations (HMO's) provide pre-paid healthcare to members of the plan. Doctors that participate with an HMO are usually paid a flat Per Member Per Month (PMPM) fee for all members. This arrangement is referred to as capitation. For example, if an insurance carrier determines that an HMO doctor would be paid $20.00 per member per month and he has 100 members, he would receive a check every month for $2000.00.

Since members lose, drop or change coverage very frequently, the PMPM amount could change every month. Although HMO doctors are not being paid on a per service basis, they are still required to bill claims as they normally would. Health insurance carriers use this data to gauge a doctor's overall managed care performance.

Managed care is a balancing act; the key is to provide quality care that is cost effective. Doctors that do not follow strict managed care practices may end up costing the plan money.

Member's that sign up with an HMO plan will be assigned a primary doctor, referred to as a Primary Care Physician (PCP). The PCP's role is to act as a gatekeeper. They will determine the most appropriate level of care based on the patient's condition.

Patients with minor illnesses, injuries, or controlled conditions, may be treated on a lower, less costly, level of care. This means minimal follow-up visits and fewer diagnostic tests. Patients with chronic or serious illnesses or injuries may require a more extensive, more expensive, level of care. This means regular follow-up visits, more diagnostic tests and more specialized care.

Members are attracted to HMO's primarily because of the limited out-of-pocket expenses. In lieu of deductibles and co-insurance amounts, members pay a flat per visit co-payment, usually between $5.00-$25.00. Members should always consult their benefit booklets as additional upfront costs may be required for certain services, for example, allergy tests or certain outpatient surgeries.

Out of network services are not covered under an HMO plan. Most HMO networks include a large panel of providers, of all specialties, that are able to perform a wide range of services. If a service is not available in network, a referral and preauthorization/preapproval will be required, in advance of service, before any out of network services will be paid.

Once you accept the authorization provided by the HMO, you agree not to balance bill the patient for any amounts outside of a patient's coinsurance, copay or deductible. Any other amounts must be written off.

HMOs can be organized in several ways. The most common are Staff model and Group model.

Staff Model- All doctors work for the HMO and all care is received at a central facility or location. Kaiser is set up this way.

Group Model- Doctors maintain their own practices. At the time of enrollment, members select a doctor's office or Independent Provider Association (IPA) and a Primary Care Physician (PCP). Members usually receive care at the PCP's office.

EXAMPLE OF AN HMO PLAN DESIGN

$10.00 PER VISIT COPAY

PLAN PAYS 100% FOR SERVICES PERFORMED BY HMO PROVIDERS.

NO OUT OF NETWORK BENEFITS

In this example, the patient would only have to pay $10.00 each time she sees an HMO doctor. The plan does not provide any coverage for services not performed by HMO doctors.

ADVANTAGES & DISADVANTAGES OF HMO PLANS

Advantages to Members Participating in HMO Plans

- Patients can generally receive quality care for little out of pocket costs.

Disadvantages to Members Participating in HMO Plans

- Patients do not have the freedom to go outside of an HMO network.

Advantages to Providers Participating in HMO Plans

- May result in greater, more consistent income.

Disadvantages to Providers Participating in HMO Plans

- Doctors may have to adhere to the HMO's way of treating patients. As they may not have the final decision on what kind of care may or may not be provided.

POINT OF SERVICE

A Point of Service plan provides the financial benefits of an HMO with the freedom of a PPO.

Point of Service simply means that the patient has the option, at the time services are needed, to use the HMO side of the plan, the PPO side of the plan or they can choose to select a provider that is out of network.

A Point of Service plan can function like an HMO in the sense that a patient can choose to receive care, from preventative services to specialty care, from providers that are enrolled under the HMO portion of the plan. When HMO providers are used, the patient will incur little, if any, out of pocket costs; in most cases just a copay.

HMO plans are restrictive by limiting access to the HMO panel of doctors only; with no coverage for any out of network services. The plan will include a large team of in network providers, from all specialties, in which to choose from.

Point of Service plans can also function like PPO plans. The patient is not restricted to using only in network providers. They have the freedom to see any provider they choose, in or out of network, no referral required, as long as they are willing to pay the increased out of pocket costs.

So maybe a patient with a POS plan hears about a great new dermatologist across town that is not in their HMO network but they may be a part of their PPO network or they could even be out of network. Here lies the true beauty of a Point of Service plan, this patient could decide to be treated by this dermatologist and have all medically necessary services covered and paid for at the in network or out of network benefit level (depending on the patient's insurance). The patient may or may not end up paying more out of pocket, but nothing beats having the freedom to choose.

With a Point of Service plan a patient can continue to see an HMO provider for treatment of high blood pressure, have weekly chiropractic visits by an in network PPO provider and arrange to see that great out of network dermatologist all at the same time.

EXAMPLE OF A POS PLAN

LEVEL 1 - HMO PLAN:	LEVEL 2 - PPO PLAN:	LEVEL 3 - OUT OF NETWORK
BENEFITS	BENEFITS	BENEFITS
$5.00 PER VISIT COPAY	$10.00 PER VISIT COPAY	$150.00 DEDUCTIBLE
PLAN PAYS 100% FOR SERVICES PERFORMED BY HMO PROVIDERS	PLAN PAYS 90%	PLAN PAYS 70%
NO OUT OF NETWORK BENEFITS	PATIENT PAYS 10%	PATIENT PAYS 30%
	NOTE: PATIENT CANNOT BE BILLED FOR CHARGES OVER THE CONTRACTED RATES	STOP LOSS - $3000 OF COVERED CHARGES THEN $100%
		NOTE: PATIENT IS RESPONSIBLE FOR ALL CHARGES OVER THE ALLOWED AMOUNT.

Providers that participate under Point of Service plans can be reimbursed by capitation, contracted rate, fee for service or any other methodology as determined by the carrier.

ADVANTAGES & DISADVANTAGES OF POS PLANS

Advantages to Members Participating in POS Plans

- Greater freedom to choose by whom and where to have services rendered.
- The ability to pull the highest benefit from the plan by using all levels at the same time, if needed.
- The ability to have access to specialized, maybe even holistic care, with some level of reimbursement forthcoming.

Disadvantages to Members Participating in POS Plans

- Low reimbursement for out of network providers means more out of a member's pocket.

Advantages to Providers Participating in POS Plans

- Access to a larger volume of new patients.
- More control over healthcare decisions.

Disadvantages to Providers Participating in POS Plans

- Reimbursement may not be adequate enough to justify the increase in patients.

FEE FOR SERVICE

A Fee for Service plan is one of the many types of health plans that are offered by health insurance carriers. A Fee for Service plan is the most simplistic of all of the plan types since standard Fee for Service plans are not considered managed care plans.

The patient is seen by any doctor they choose. There are no provider directories to look through in order to locate an in network provider.

- No referral or any pre-approvals are needed.
- The claims are billed to the health carrier but there is no need to try and figure out allowed amounts or contracted rates because regardless of what the health carrier ultimately pays toward that claim, the balance is deemed to be the patient's liability.

Most health carriers will not pay off the billed amount, the claim will usually pass through some type of pricing data. Usually for Fee for Service plans, that data is Usual, Customary and Reasonable (UCR).

Let's look at an example.

Dr. Smith performs an office visit for $200.00 and a chest x-ray for $100.00 and he bills the claim to the insurance company for his normal rate of $300.00. In spite of the fact that no in network arrangement exists, the health carrier will still seek ways to price this claim. After being priced, the health carrier determines that $150.00 for the office visit and $50.00 for the x-ray is accepted. The plan allows $200.00 instead of the billed amount of $300.00. The patient is responsible for the difference.

Since Fee for Service plans were written so that the plan participants would share in the cost of healthcare, members are required to pay the deductible and co-insurance amounts.

EXAMPLE OF AN FFS PLAN

Let's look at another example of how a payment would be made on a standard fee for service plan.

PLAN TYPE - FFS:

$100.00 DEDUCTIBLE

COINSURANCE PLAN PAYS 80%

PATIENT PAYS 20%

OUT OF POCKET - $5000
IN COVERED CHARGES

James has a Fee for Service plan. He becomes ill and is seen in the emergency room. His total bill is $3500.00.

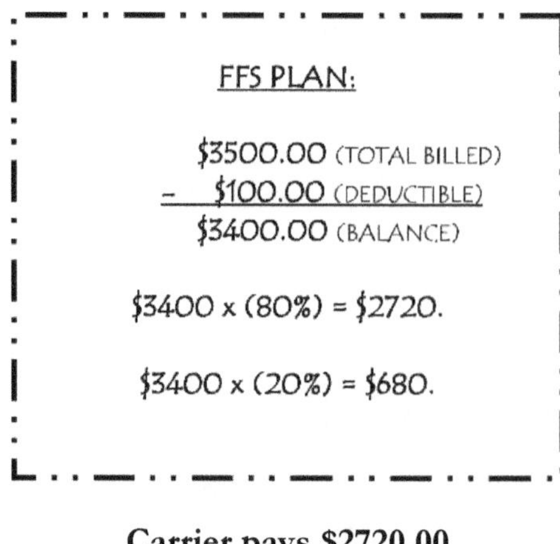

Carrier pays $2720.00

Patient pays $780.00 ($100.00 deductible + $680.00)

Standard Fee for Service plans are the most expensive plans to purchase because they do not have the managed care component that helps to control costs such as contracted providers that accept reduced rates or more front end controls and requirements.

Note: For the purpose of this article, Standard Fee for Service means that the Fee for Service plan is not part of a managed care plan.

ADVANTAGES & DISADVANTAGES OF FFS PLANS

Advantages to Members Participating in FFS Plans

- Members have the freedom to select any doctor and not worry about in network or out of network.
- They can see any doctor or specialist without having to wait for a referral or preapproval.
- Plan is easier to understand and out of pocket is easy to predict. Usually a flat percentage of billed will be expected on all charges.

Disadvantages to Members Participating in FFS Plans

- The member can expect to pay more out of pocket because the provider is not required to accept the health carrier's allowed amounts. The provider can bill what he wants and make the patient responsible for any amounts not paid by insurance.
- Due to the unpredictability of UCR rates, a member will not be able to determine how much their health carrier will pay for a service.
- Higher premium costs.

Advantages to Providers Participating in FFS Plans

- Providers can expect a flat percentage of costs.
- No need to worry about which methodology will be used to calculate the claim.
- Plan will be easier to understand.
- Patients can be billed for any non-covered charges.

Disadvantages to Providers Participating in FFS Plans

- Very few employers choose FFS plans resulting in fewer patients with FFS plans.

COMMERCIAL PLANS

Companies like Humana, Prudential, Cigna and Aetna are considered commercial health insurance carriers. This means they are in the business of writing and selling health insurance plans that provide coverage for medical services, treatment and supplies.

Health plans that are written by commercial health carriers come in a wide range of different plan designs and plan types:

- From HMO to Fee-for-Service plans.
- From no deductible and no coinsurance to high deductible and high coinsurance.
- From traditional to managed care plans.

Most core features can be customized to fit the employer's needs and their budget. Because plan designs could differ greatly by carrier, it is possible that two different members that share the same commercial carrier may have two entirely separate benefit plan designs.

For Example:

Susan Smith works for ABC Company and has a PPO health insurance plan with Aetna and James Jones works for XYZ Company and also has a PPO health insurance plan with Aetna.

Susan's plan was written to provide for office visits with only a $5.00 copay if she picks a doctor that is in her network. James is required to pay a $100.00 deductible for all in network services.

Just because two patients share the same carrier, you cannot assume that benefits are the same. You will always need to contact the carrier to verify benefits.

Each commercial carrier has a list of plans that they offer and the hope is that an employer or an insurance agent working on behalf of an employer, will be persuaded to choose one commercial carrier over another. The Insurance Agent's role is to do the legwork that most employers do not have the time to do.

For Example

Joe's Carpet Cleaning is a new company with 25 employees and they are looking for health insurance for the group. The employer could contact each commercial health carrier himself but most likely he will use an Insurance Agent. Think of an insurance agent like a real estate agent.

Let's say you decide that you want to buy a house. So you contact a real estate agent, give them a list of your "must haves," like location, size and price, and let them get busy. The Agent's job is to find that best fit. Well this process is about the same for employers that are looking for health insurance. The Insurance Agent will look at all of the health carriers: Cigna, Humana, etc., to find the one that best fits the employer's list of must haves.

The Agent will present his list of good candidates to the employer for review and selection. If all goes as planned, the employer will enroll with one of the carriers on the list, the employees will get the health insurance they need and the insurance agent will get a commission.

Commercial health carriers are also in the business of administering the plans that they write. Once the sale is completed, the real work begins as the carrier is expected to handle all aspects of the insurance process including:

- Enrollment
- Issuing ID cards
- Collecting premiums
- Processing claims
- Enrolling providers
- Updating provider directories
- Issuing Summary Plan Descriptions or plan booklets
- Handling appeals and disputes

Most commercial health insurance carriers also administer state Medicaid plans and some Medicare managed care plans. As you can see, the business of health insurance is not unlike any other business. Commercial health insurance carriers need to remain competitive in order to retain the customers they have and they need a constant flow of new accounts to keep them in business.

MEDICAID

Medicaid is a federal program that provides health coverage for low-income families with children, low-income elderly, and disabled people. The federal government and each state share in the cost of Medicaid programs. Each state sets their own perimeters for eligibility which is mostly based on one's ability to pay for healthcare.

Because Medicaid has strict requirements that must be followed in order to remain eligible for coverage, Medicaid coverage could change from eligible to not eligible from month to month. Make sure you check eligibility for each visit.

The Medicaid program has recently expanded eligibility to 133% of the poverty level. This was because of the Affordable Care Act's requirement that all must have health insurance or incur a penalty. Children under the age of 21 could also qualify for added coverage under one of their state's Special Children's Services programs.

Medicaid plans can be administered by the state, meaning that the state has a separate department that is tasked with the handling of claim related services, including claim processing. Medicaid plans can also be administered by a health insurance carrier, like Blue Cross Blue Shield or United Healthcare, who is acting on the state's behalf by processing claims for patients with Medicaid.

Medicaid plans normally have some type of pre-authorization requirements which could vary by Medicaid carrier. Some requirements include:

1. Pre-approval for all services over a stated dollar amount. For example, all services over $500.00.

2. Pre-approval by procedure. For example, all CT scans or DME supplies.

3. All services require pre-authorization.

All pre approval requirements must be completed before the patient comes in the office. Most Medicaid plans will not allow a retrospective request; a request for approval after the service was rendered.

Providers who choose to participate with Medicaid agree to abide by the rules as set forth by the plan and they agree to accept the Medicaid payment as payment in full. Of course, they can expect patients to pay for any copayments (this is rare) or not covered charges.

Medicaid patients cannot be balance billed for any amounts not deemed patient liability.

Medicaid does not have a standard way to administer their plans. This means don't expect that all states operate exactly the same:

- Every state has some discretion in the way care is delivered, claims are processed and payments are made.

- Medicaid plans could range from a Fee For Service plan to a Managed Care plan.
- Plans could be administered by the state or they could use a health carrier to handle all claim related issues, enrollments, and claim payments.
- Plan members have the option to choose a traditional fee for service plan or any of the different managed care plans like a PPO or an HMO.

Reimbursement could also range greatly from one state to the next. For example, Medicaid reimbursement is higher in California than it is in Louisiana because the cost to live in California is more expensive. Cost of living is one of the many factors that are used to come up with this pricing data.

Medicaid covered services include:

- In and outpatient hospital charges
- Prenatal care
- Doctor's services
- Lab and x-ray services
- Well child care under 21 years old
- Family planning
- Home health care and nursing facilities
- Other coverages like vision, eyeglasses, prescription drugs, dental, etc., may be available depending upon funding.

Medicaid Eligibility

Medicaid members must first meet the financial requirements in order to qualify for coverage. Those with lower incomes, the unemployed, dependent children or those with a disability may more easily meet the Medicaid parameters for coverage, but those that are employed can also be deemed eligible.

Even if a person's income exceeds Medicaid's requirements that person may be able to qualify for coverage under Medicaid Spend Down. Medicaid Spend Down allows you to use existing medical bills as a way to help qualify for Medicaid coverage.

Spend Down is available only to those:

- Persons under 21
- Persons over 65
- Disabled or blind
- In some situations where a parent is absent, out of work or deceased.

Once it is determined how much excess income a person has, they can use medical bills to offset the excess.

For Example

It is determined that a person's income is over the Medicaid requirement by $450.00 but they have just spent $500.00 for new glasses. They can apply this $500.00 to reduce the $450.00 excess income so they would now be eligible for Medicaid coverage for that month. Of course, if eligibility is solely based on spend down, you must repeat this process every month.

The ability to spend down to obtain Medicaid coverage may be critical for some patients with serious health conditions and only one health plan leaving them responsible for the huge medical bills.

Most states now provide online access to Medicaid eligibility verifications, claim status, Remittance Advice/EOB's, pre authorization requests and even a claim payment system where you can bill claims directly. Simply complete the enrollment process at the state Medicaid website.

MEDICARE

Medicare is a federal health insurance program that provides health insurance coverage for members, called beneficiaries. Medicare applies to beneficiaries who are 65 or older and are citizens or permanent residents of the United States, certain younger people with disabilities or anyone who has end stage renal disease.

We have a tendency to separate Medicare into two categories - Traditional Medicare and Medicare Managed Care. The benefits, processes, rules and procedures differ greatly between the two.

Medicare beneficiaries may receive:

1. Medicare Part A - Hospital coverage that pays for hospital services, skilled nursing facilities, home health and hospice care. There is no cost to most beneficiaries. It is based on years in the work force.
2. Medicare Part B - Medical, professional or traditional coverage as it pays for doctor's services, outpatient therapy, durable medical equipment, supplies and other needed services. Monthly premium payment is required.
3. Medicare Part C - Part of Medicare Part B. It is not really a separate coverage rather it allows for beneficiaries to select a managed care plan instead of a traditional 80/20 plan.
4. Medicare Part D Prescription Drug - This provides coverage for prescription drugs. This coverage is optional and requires payment of an additional premium.

Medicare beneficiaries have several options to change coverage from one plan type to another. This is why, especially at the beginning of each year, you should verify coverage for each encounter.

Medicare Enrollment

Once you are approaching age 65, you will have a 7 month enrollment period in which to enroll for Medicare coverage. You have up to 3 months prior to the month of your birth, the month of your birth, up until 3 months after in which to enroll. If you miss this period, you will have to wait until the next scheduled open enrollment period.

Disabled persons are eligible to enroll for Medicare once they have been on SSI for 24 months.

After enrollment is completed, the beneficiary will receive a Red, White and Blue ID card. The beneficiary's ID number is their 9-digit social security number, plus a one or two-digit suffix (added to back of the ID number, ex. 123456789A). A description of some of these suffixes is described below:

1. A WAGE EARNER
2. D AGED WIDOW
3. B AGED WIFE
4. D4 REMARRIED WIDOW
5. B1 HUSBAND
6. E MOTHER (WIDOW)

7. C1 CHILDREN

8. F1 FATHER

9. F2 MOTHER

Note: In keeping with the HIPAA requirement that all patient's PHI (Protected Health Information) must be kept secure, the social security number listed on all Medicare ID cards must be replaced with an encrypted number before 2019.

Medicare Managed Care vs. Medicare Traditional

- Medicare Traditional plans, normally, do not require preapproval or preauthorization for certain medical services and surgery. Medicare coverage policies are located online and they provide full details on the procedures, parameters for coverage, the associated codes, etc. As long as the patient fits the criteria for coverage, they can proceed.
- Medicare Managed care plans usually require some level of preapproval or preauthorization for certain medical services and surgery.
- Medicare Fee Schedule provides reimbursement amounts for a just about every service, treatment or supply. Beneficiaries with traditional Medicare will have a general idea of what, if any, costs they can expect to incur.
- Medicare Managed care plans can be reimbursed under the Medicare Fee Schedule, by contracted rate, capitation or any other type of methodology.
- Traditional Medicare plans pay 80% of allowed. The beneficiary is responsible for the 20% or it can be billed to a Medigap plan.

- Medicare Managed care plans could have a host of different plans and benefits. The managed care plan must provide the same level of coverage that would be available under the traditional plan or better.
- Providers that participate with Medicare traditional plans, agree to accept the Medicare assignment. This means that they agree to accept the Medicare allowed amount and can only bill the patient for any applicable coinsurance or deductible.
- Providers that opt out or chose not to participate with Medicare can only collect up to 115% of the limiting charge plus 20% as well as any applicable deductible.
- All providers are required, by law, to submit claims for Medicare Beneficiaries and they cannot bill the patient for a claim filing fee.

Medicare does not pay for:

- Custodial care
- Nursing home care
- Full-time nursing care in the home
- Dental care and dentures
- Most eyeglasses and eye exams or routine physical exams/checkups (except screening Pap smears and screening mammograms)
- Most immunization shots (except the pneumonia vaccine, flu vaccine and Hepatitis B vaccine)
- Over-the-counter drugs
- Routine foot care
- Hearing aids or the tests associated with them
- Private duty nurses
- Extra charges for a private room
- Personal comfort items

- Cosmetic surgery
- Any chiropractic service, except for treatment of subluxation of the spine and services considered not reasonable and necessary.

Medicare states that:

- During the first 45 days of coverage, Medicare beneficiaries can change from a Managed Care Plan to an original (traditional) Medicare plan.
- Beneficiaries with original (traditional) Medicare cannot switch to a Managed Care Plan.
- Beneficiaries cannot change from one Managed Care to another.
- Beneficiaries can change plans during Open Enrollment which is October 15-December 15.

RAILROAD MEDICARE

Railroad Medicare is program that provides health insurance coverage to retirees, survivors, families and some workers with permanent disabilities. One must have worked 10 or more years with the railroad service to be eligible for coverage.

Railroad Medicare provides the same basic coverage that is provided by the federal Medicare program, including:

Part A- includes doctors services, laboratory services, outpatient hospital services, Home Health Care Services.

Part B – includes physicians and other services not paid under Part A.

Railroad Medicare Enrollment

The Railroad Retirement Board is responsible for the enrollment and collection of premiums which are usually deducted monthly.

After enrollment is completed, the beneficiary will receive a red, white and blue ID card that clearly states Railroad Retirement Board across the front. The beneficiary's ID number will be a 6 or 9 digit number with a

1, 2, or 3-digit prefix (added to front of the ID number, ex. A123456789). A description of some of these prefixes are described below:

1. A Railroad Retiree – file established when the employee was alive.
2. MA Spouse of the Railroad Retiree.
3. MH Spouse of the Railroad Retiree
4. H Employee on Railroad pension when Act passed in 1937
5. WA Widow (er) of the retiree – file established when the employee was alive.
6. WH Widow(er) – employee on Railroad pension when Act passed in 1937.
7. WD Widow(er) of the retiree – file established after the retiree deceased.
8. WCA Disabled child of the retiree – file established while the retiree was alive.

Note: The ID card issued by the Federal Government is also red, white and blue but it displays Social Security Medicare across the front and the number has a suffix not a prefix- meaning the alpha is place at the end for federal Medicare and the Beginning for Railroad.

In a Nutshell

Railroad Medicare claims are handled just like you would any other Medicare claim except that claims are billed directly to Palmetto GBA. Visit www.palmettogba.com for more information.

MEDIGAP

When a patient enrolls in Medicare, they have the option to choose either:

A Traditional Medicare plan - which is an 80/20 plan. Medicare pays 80% of the Medicare allowed amount and the patient is responsible for paying 20% of the Medicare allowed amount.

OR

A Medicare Managed Care plan - which could include a wide range of variations in plan designs. Most Medicare plans are HMO, PPO or FFS plans where reimbursement could range from being paid in full, after a copay, (like an HMO plan) to 80% or less (like a PPO plan).

Some Medicare patients (called beneficiaries) may choose not to enroll in a managed care plan in spite of the possible higher level of reimbursement and the lower out of pocket costs, for a lot of reasons:

- Maybe the provider that they love and trust is not part of the managed care network.
- Maybe the cost for a managed care plan is too high.
- Maybe they refuse to surrender their right to choose the providers they want to see.

Whatever the reason, quite a few Medicare beneficiaries still choose Medicare traditional plans.

Medigap polices, also called Medicare Supplemental Plans, were designed for this group of Medicare beneficiaries as a way to prevent them from incurring financial hardship due to the 20% portion deemed to be patient responsibility. Medigap policies are a second health plan that can be purchased to help bridge that gap in coverage.

The Medigap plan will pick up 20% of what Medicare allows leaving the patient, in most cases, with a little more than the plan deductible to pay out of pocket. Some Medigap plans will even pick up the plan deductible.

In a nutshell, Medigap is…

- Private insurance coverage that is offered to Medicare beneficiaries who have Part A (hospital) and Part B (professional).
- Coverage which can be purchased from any insurance carrier that is licensed in the state.
- Coverage with a separate premium to the insurance carrier that must be paid in addition to the Part B premium.
- A policy that cannot be canceled as long as the premium is paid; even if the beneficiary has serious health problems.
- A plan that will kick in after Medicare pays and may provide reimbursement for the deductible and 20% coinsurance that is not paid for by Medicare.
- A big plus for beneficiaries that choose the traditional Medicare plans, as it will severely limit the money that seniors will have to pay out of their pocket for healthcare.
- A plan that may not be necessary for beneficiaries that choose one of the managed care plans because managed care plans are designed to limit a patient's out of pocket expense as long as in-network providers are used.
- Available in 10 different plan types and are designed to provide a wide range of coverages including:

basic medical, preventative, hospital or skilled nursing, to name a few. The beneficiary can pick the Medigap plan that best fits their needs.

- Not mandatory. A Medicare beneficiary may choose to enroll in a traditional Medicare plan, forgo the Medigap plan and just pay the 20% out of pocket. It is totally up to the Medicare beneficiary to decide.

MILITARY

Tricare, formerly known as Champus, is the health plan that is available to the brave service men and women (and their families) that protect our country.

Initially, people in the military were required to go to a designated military facility for medical services and treatment. Due to issues with these facilities, including limited number of facilities and overcrowding, this requirement was changed sometime in the 1980's when the program was restructured to mirror the way health plans are administrated by health insurance companies.

This restructuring included:

- Direct access to any of the hundreds of providers that will accept the Tricare allowed amounts.
- Internal departments that would handle the enrollment, premium collection and claim processing services.
- Redesigned health plans to include the cost containment features of a managed care plan.

This simplification and expanded access to care made it much easier for our military heroes and their families to receive the care they need.

Military members and their families can choose one of the numerous health plans based on the category they fall in. Some of the categories are:

- Active duty and their families
- Active National Guard/Reserve and their families
- Survivors
- Children
- Qualified Former spouses
- Medal of Honor Recipients
- Retired service members and their families
- Missing in action

Military and their families have several different plan types available to them depending on their status. Some of these plan types include:

- TRICARE Prime, Remote and Overseas - this plan is available to active duty members and their families and well as other categories of service members and their families. This plan is a zero cost plan as long as in network providers are used. No premiums, no deductibles, no copays, and no out of pocket costs. This plan is similar to an HMO plan where members are assigned a Primary Care Physician and directed to participating providers. This plan also has a Point of Service component where out of network providers can be used at out of pocket costs.
- TRICARE Standard, Extra and Overseas - this plan is available to active duty members and their families as well as other categories of service members and their families. This plan works like a PPO plan where in network or out of network providers can be used.
- TRICARE for Life – Available to military members who have Medicare part A and Part B. This plan works like a Medigap plan were the Tricare plan will pay only after Medicare has paid its portion.

- TRICARE Reserve Select – Available to Qualified Selected Reserve members and their families. This plan works like a PPO plan, in network or out of network providers can be used. Members pay the annual premium, plan deductibles and coinsurance amounts.
- TRICARE Retired Reserve – Available to qualified retired reserve members and their families and survivors of retired reserve members. This plan works like a PPO plan where in network or out of network providers can be used. Members pay the annual premium, plan deductibles and coinsurance amounts.
- TRICARE Young Adult- For adult dependents of eligible service men and women that are age 21-26. Premiums are required.
- US Family Health Plan - Available to active duty members and their families and well as others categories of service members and their families who live in designed areas.

In a nutshell

Military service members have a lot of different health plan options based on what category they fall into. But there is no need to worry, all of this has been sorted out by the time they reach the provider's office.

The ID card will be the first step to finding out the plan, eligibility and benefits that are available – in other words you will handle this plan just as you would every other health plan.

WORKERS COMPENSATION

When an employee is injured on the job, the way that they would access medical care for a work related injury is totally different from the way they would access medical care for a non-work related injury.

For example…

Jane Z. slips and falls on the stairway at work and injures her right shoulder. She is still able to work, but she is in pain. Her plan was to go see her primary care physician on the way home from work, but she is growing more concerned and not really sure what she should do. Her injury is work related yet she is worried about filing a work comp claim.

What should Jane do?

Jane should first notify her employer about the injury. She would then be asked to file a claim that provides a detailed account of the accident, including:

- When the injury occurred.
- What part of the body is injured.
- Date and time of injury.

- How it happened.
- Where it happened.
- Any conditions that may have contributed to the injury, slippery, wet, icy etc.

The employer would then refer her to a medical provider to be checked out. The provider would interview her, perform a full exam and detail her injuries. Depending on her injuries, she may be released to return to work unrestricted, with restrictions, or, in some cases, the condition may be severe enough that she may be unable to return to work. She would then be managed by a Workers Compensation approved provider until released from care.

Workers Compensation guarantees:

- Replacement of loss wages
- Medical care
- Rehabilitation
- Other benefits

What is Workers Compensation?

Workers Compensation is required by each state and is insurance coverage that all employers are required to purchase. The purpose is to provide coverage to employees that become ill or injured as a result of their job.

Employers pay premiums to a state fund and claims are handled by the insurance carrier. Each state administers its own program. Claims are filed by the employer to the insurance carrier, who then files with the state.

Workers can receive lost wages and coverage for medical care, dismemberment, disability and death. Workers can go to the assigned doctor or they can request to have an Independent Medical Exam (IME) performed by a doctor of their choice. The doctor will examine the sick or injured worker to determine the condition, the degree of disability and if and when the worker can return to work. Workers compensation plans pay primary to any other health plan.

So why does this matter?

It matters because seeing a patient that has an open workers compensation case, unless the provider has clear authorization to treat, may result in nonpayment of the claim.

Most group plans do not provide coverage for any work related illness or injury.

Patients that seek treatment for some specific conditions or complaints such as back pain, accidents and injuries should be queried about how the condition occurred. Sometimes a patient will seek care from a non-work approved provider because they are reluctant to file a claim for fear of retaliation or loss of job.

Every state has a Worker Compensation Board with detailed information that can be found online. Patients with unreported injuries should be referred to the website for help with the process.

BLUE CROSS BLUE SHIELD

Blue Cross Blue Shield (BCBS) is known as one of the largest health insurance carriers in the nation, but Blue Cross Blue Shield is more than that. It is actually a group of individual companies that joined together to contract with healthcare providers to provide care to its plan members.

Think of Blue Cross Blue Shield like one big umbrella, under which stands a host of different companies, all using the Blue Cross Blue Shield name. Some examples include:

- Blue Cross Blue Shield
- Regence Blue Cross Blue Shield
- Empire Blue Cross Blue Shield
- Highmark Blue Cross Blue Shield
- Anthem Blue Cross Blue Shield
- Premera Blue Cross Blue Shield
- All the various state Blue Cross Blue Shields like BCBS of AL, BCBS of MN, BCBS of IL, etc.

Blue Cross refers mainly to plans for hospital services and outpatient care. Blue Shield refers mainly to plans for doctor's services. In some states, BCBS is together as one company and in other states, like California for one, Blue Cross operates separately from Blue Shield.

So why does this matter?

In truth, this really does not matter at all because Blue Cross Blue Shield functions just like any other health insurance carrier. Some of these functions include:

- Writing of health insurance plans.
- Selling of health insurance plans.
- Administering health insurance plans.
- Processing claims.

Key features of BCBS

BCBS has numerous different plan designs from HMO to FFS and everything in between. They also administer some Medicare and Medicaid plans.

Blue Cross Blue Shield has an impressive provider network. It is hard to find a provider that is not associated with at least one of the Blue Cross Blue Shield plans. Providers who contract with BCBS plans, depending on the plan type, agree to provide care at discounted or contracted rates in exchange for access to more patients. Due to the fact that Blue Cross Blue Shield insures hundreds of thousands of lives, the expectation of having access to more patients may be realized.

In a nutshell

Blue Cross Blue Shield is most likely the carrier that you will work with the most often due to the number of members that have a Blue Cross Blue Shield plan.

Don't be fooled into thinking that just because the name is the same that everything else is the same.

The name may be the same, but they are not a one-size-fits-all carrier. Every state could differ. The plans, processes and procedures could differ. The benefits, plans and coverages could differ. Take the time to verify coverage on all patients.

Unlike other health carriers, the member ID located on the patient's ID card, with its alpha numeric numbering system makes it easy to tell at a glance that you are working with a Blue Cross Blue Shield plan.

Subscribers are given a unique BCBS ID number that has a plan-specific alpha three-digit prefix, with up to 14 digits after - example ZAP123456789121. The first two characters of the prefix identify each plan and the third character identifies the type of product the subscriber is enrolled in.

BCBS also administers plans for employees of the federal government. Their ID cards for federal employees (FEP) do not have a three-digit alpha prefix. These ID numbers begin with the letter "R."

MANAGED CARE PLAN

A Managed Care Plan is a plan that is designed to manage how healthcare is delivered to a patient in an effort to control costs.

This is accomplished in a lot of different ways, including:

- Primary care providers
- Referrals
- Preapprovals
- Copays
- Coinsurance
- Deductibles
- In network providers
- No out of network coverage

For Patients

Managed care plans provide patients access to a wide network of providers at lower out of pocket costs. This makes a managed care plan ideal. Especially for patients/families that are healthy or have controlled conditions that only require the lowest levels of care.

For patients with complex health issues, gaining access to alternative or specialized levels of care may be a slow process. You may have to wait to exhaust some lower levels of care first or the plan may have a referral and authorization requirement that delays care.

Most plans today are written as managed care plans, but the attractiveness of the lower out of pocket cost should be weighed against the inability to access any provider that you want unless you are willing to pay more out of pocket.

Real World Example

For the last few years, someone I know has suffered from a host of uncomfortable, though not life threatening, illnesses i.e. stomach issues, rashes, itching, etc. I believe her Primary Care Physician described them as "nuisance issues." Because she had an HMO plan, she was required to stay in the network. In spite of the numerous visits and prescriptions, she only experienced temporary relief.

She decided to pay out of her own pocket to see a holistic specialist that she was recommended to. The cost for the visit and extensive lab work was pricey but she discovered that her condition was related to food allergies.

She swears she is 100% better and even swapped out her HMO plan so that she could at least have some out of network coverage.

This example illustrates what some say is wrong with some managed care plans. Because no one can predict health, having the freedom to go outside of the circle without having to pay an arm and two legs for it - is important; especially for situations of repeat visits with no improvement.

For Providers

The appeal of managed care contracts is evident - an increase in patients results in a steady stream of income. Besides, what doctor today can afford to opt out of all of the managed care plans? Participation has become almost mandatory. Providers that sign managed care contracts just need to fully understand what it may mean to their practice.

The payment methodology should be clear. Will you have upfront access to the reimbursement amounts for your most common procedures so you can determine loss or gain? Can you appeal payments with an outside reviewer? Will claims be paid promptly?

My thoughts

You can choose to participate with every health carrier nationwide, but if you are not managing your operation it is not going to give you the result you are looking for which is an increase in revenue. Here are some musts before signing on the dotted line with any carrier:

- Thoroughly review all contracts before you sign.
- Keep your eye on all claim's payments to make sure that you are being reimbursed as expected.
- Make sure you appeal or dispute every claim that is paid incorrectly.
- Review all contracts periodically to make sure they are really worth it.
- If the talent needed to recover every dime that is due does not exist in your practice - outsource.

There is nothing worse than getting stuck with low reimbursement with little or no chance to renegotiate the contract in exchange for a few new patients.

Please note that portions of this article reflect my opinions and experiences only. Use this as yet another source of information.

CHAPTER TWO TEST

Directions: Using what you have learned in Chapter Two, answer the following questions.

1. Are plan members covered under a PPO plan allowed to use out of network providers?

2. What does exclusive mean in reference to EPO plans?

3. What is PMPM mean in HMO plans?

4. Which is more restrictive an HMO or a POS? Explain.

5. Does a FFS plan provide the greatest benefit to the plan member or the provider?

6. What is a commercial health plan?

7. A managed care plan's primary role is to?

8. What does spend down mean?

9. What is a 7 month enrollment period?

10. Is a Medicare beneficiary required to take a Medigap plan?

11. Tricare was formally referred to by what name?

12. Why does it matter if a patient comes in with a work related injury?

13. What is unique about the Blue Cross Blue Shield ID numbers?

3 BENEFITS & PROVISIONS

Chapter Overview - Every health plan is written to provide a long list of benefits and provisions. The key is to understand how these benefits will affect the bottom line. In this chapter, we will show you how benefits really work.

This Chapter Includes:

Individual Deductible

Family Deductible

Out of Pocket

Copay

Coinsurance

Participating Provider

Non-Participating Provider

Primary Care Physician

ID Card

Summary Plan Description

Consolidated Omnibus Budget Reconciliation Act

Utilization Review

Referral

Eligibility

Subrogation

Letter of Agreement

Gap Exception

Medical Necessity

INDIVIDUAL DEDUCTIBLE

Most health insurance plans are written with the expectation that all plan members must share in the cost of providing healthcare coverage. A deductible is the portion of the claim that the patient will be required to pay before the insurance carrier will pay anything. The deductible starts over every year.

Let's use sample ABC plan for our first example of how the individual deductible is applied.

JAMES' ABC PLAN:

$300.00 Individual Deductible

$900.00 Family Deductible

$3000.00 Max Out of Pocket

80% In Network

50% Out of Network

Visit 1

James E. is a member of ABC plan. He is seen by the doctor and incurs $200.00 in health care costs. Since none of his deductible is met, he is required to pay the full $200.00 upfront.

The claim for $200.00 is submitted to his health plan. They allow the full $200.00 and apply it to his plan deductible thus paying zero.

Visit 2

James is seen again by his provider and again his bill is $200.00. Because he already met $200.00 of a $300.00 deductible, the provider requires he pay $100.00 plus 20% (his plan pays at 80%).

The claim for $200.00 is submitted to his health plan. They allow the full $200.00 and apply $100.00 to his plan deductible. The other $100.00 is paid at 80%.

Visit 3

James is seen for one final visit but this bill is only for $100.00. Because his deductible is met in full, James is required to pay 20% only.

The claim for $100.00 is submitted to his health plan. They allow the full $100.00 and since his deductible is met in full, his plan reimburses 80% to the provider.

The deductible is all about timing. For example…

Mr. Smith is in the office and his health carrier is called to verify eligibility and benefits. We learn that he has an 80/20 PPO plan with a $250.00 deductible. None of his $250.00 plan deductible has been met for this year. Mr. Smith insists that because he saw his Chiropractor three times last week, his deductible is now met, in full. We apologize, explain our policy for upfront payment and assure him that after the claim is processed, if a refund is due it will be handled immediately. He unhappily pulls out his credit card and is charged $250.00 plus his 20% coinsurance amount.

He sees the doctor, incurs $500.00 in charges and his claim is billed to his health plan.

Although, Mr. Smith saw the chiropractor 3 times ***last*** week, how the deductible is applied is all about timing. Because our claim reached his health carrier BEFORE the claim from the chiropractor, the $250.00 deductible was taken from the claim we billed, not from the claim from the Chiropractor.

The amount he was required to pay upfront was correct and no refund was due from us. His chiropractor may owe him a refund.

The way the deductible is applied is all about timing because the deductible will be taken from the claim that is processed first. **The date of service may have nothing to do with how the deductible is applied unless the claim with the earlier date of service is processed first.**

Please note that the allowed amount is critical to understanding what amounts may be applied to the plan deductible, what may be paid and even which portion is not covered.

I discuss allowed amounts in detail in Chapter 7 - Reimbursement.

FAMILY DEDUCTIBLE

Most health insurance plans are written with the expectation that all plan members must share in the cost of providing healthcare coverage. A deductible is the portion of the claim that the patient will be required to pay before the insurance carrier will pay anything. The deductible starts over every year.

Most plans are written to include a family deductible along with the individual deductible. The family deductible is the maximum that will be applied on all family members during the current benefit year.

Let's use sample ABC plan for an example of how a family deductible is applied.

JOHN'S ABC PLAN:

$300.00 Individual Deductible

$900.00 Family Deductible

$3000.00 Max Out of Pocket

80% In Network

50% Out of Network

John and his wife Jane have three kids named Joey, Joan and Samy. Everybody comes down with the flu so everyone has to see the doctor.

- John incurs $300.00 in health care expenses. His deductible was already met on a previous claim and his plan pays at 80% of billed.
- Jane incurs $300.00 in health care expenses and her full claim is applied to the plan deductible.
- Joey incurs $100.00 in expenses and his full claim is applied to the deductible.
- Joan incurs $100.00 in expenses and her full claim is applied to the deductible
- Samy incurs $200.00 in expenses and $100.00 of his claim is applied to the deductible. The other $100.00 is paid at 80%. So the family deductible is met based on the combined accumulation of all family members.

FAMILY DEDUCTIBLE:	
JOHN	$300.00
JANE	$300.00
JOEY	$100.00
JOAN	$100.00
SAMY	$100.00
	$900.00

The $900.00 family deductible is met so no further deductible can be taken from any family members for the duration of the plan year. Without a family deductible maximum, the family of five would have incurred $1500.00, or a $300.00 per member individual deductible.

Let's look at another example using slightly different billed amounts.

- John incurs $100.00 in healthcare expenses and his full claim is applied to the plan deductible.
- Jane incurs $100.00 in health care expenses and her full claim is applied to the plan deductible.

- Joey incurs $100.00 in expenses and his full claim is applied to the deductible.
- Joan incurs $100.00 in expenses and her full claim is applied to the deductible
- Samy incurs $100.00 in expenses and his claim is applied to the deductible.

Using this second example, this family of five has already incurred $500.00 in health care expenses. NONE of it will be reimbursed by the health plan leaving the family to pay this $500.00 out of pocket. No one has met their individual deductible of $300.00 per person and the family did not meet the family deductible of $900.00. These two examples provide a general overview of how the family deductible may be applied. The way the deductible is applied is all about timing, so each experience may be different.

Please note that the allowed amount is critical to understanding what amounts may be applied to the plan deductible, what will be paid and even what portion is not covered.

I discuss allowed amounts in detail in Chapter 7 - Reimbursement.

OUT OF POCKET

Since most health plans are written to require some level of cost sharing, the Out of Pocket Maximum refers to the amount that a patient is expected to pay for healthcare. This portion will not be reimbursed by the health plan unless a patient has a secondary coverage.

Out of pocket is the maximum amount that you would have to pay out of your pocket for all covered medical services, treatment and supplies. The out of pocket maximum, or stop loss provision, is designed to keep a patient from incurring great debt due to the high cost of medical care. All claims will be paid at the plan percentage (coinsurance) until the maximum out of pocket has been reached. After that, all claims will be paid at 100% of the allowed amount for the rest of the plan year. Keep in mind that any copays, not covered amounts or any amounts that are over the allowed amount will not be included in the out of pocket maximum. A patient may still be responsible for these amounts.

Let's look at how out of pocket may work using ABC plan example.

ROBIN'S ABC PLAN:

$300.00 Individual Deductible

$900.00 Family Deductible

$3000.00 Max Out of Pocket

80% In Network

50% Out of Network

Robin J. has an emergency appendectomy and incurs a hospital bill for $20,000.00. Using the ABC plan, her carrier may reimburse the hospital claim as follows: (Let's assume that this is the first claim for this year so her deductible has not been met and that the full bill is allowed as presented)

HOSPITAL BILL:

$20,000.00
- $300.00 (DEDUCTIBLE)
$19,700.00 (BALANCE)

PATIENT WILL PAY: $3300.00
($300.00 DEDUCTIBLE + $3000.00 STOP LOSS)

CARRIER WILL PAY $16,700.00
($20,000 - $3300 PATIENT'S PORTION)

Let's look at Robin's second claim for the surgery. Robin is charged $5000.00 for the surgery. When presented to the insurance carrier, the claim will be processed in the following way. (Let's assume that the billed amount of $5000.00 has been allowed in full.)

SURGERY BILL:

$5,000.00

$5000.00 x (100%) = $5000.00

CARRIER WILL PAY: $5000.00

PATIENT WILL PAY $0.00
(THE DEDUCTIBLE AND MAX OUT OF POCKET HAS BEEN MET)

Keep in mind that every plan is different. Some plans are written to include the deductible in the maximum out of pocket. Using the hospital claim for Robin, if the deductible was included in the OOP it would be calculated like this.

HOSPITAL BILL:

$20,000.00
- $300.00 (DEDUCTIBLE INCLUDED IN OOP)
$19,700.00 (BALANCE)

PATIENT WILL PAY: $3000.00
($300.00 DEDUCTIBLE + $2700.00 STOP LOSS)

CARRIER WILL PAY $17,000.00
($20,000 - $3000 PATIENT'S PORTION)

So looking at these two examples, although the $3000.00 out of pocket is a huge amount to pay, what if her plan did not have the Out of Pocket Maximum provision?

Robin would have been responsible for roughly 20% of all allowed charges plus her plan deductible.

Total billed for the surgery and hospital charges = $25,000.00 - $300.00 deductible = $24,700

$24,700.00 x 20% = $4940.00

She would have paid $5240.00 ($4940.00 + $300.00 deductible) instead of the $3300.00 she was required to pay.

The other plus is that all claims billed during that same plan year will be paid at 100% of the allowed amount. These claims can be related or unrelated to her surgery, no matter. As long as the treatment, service or supply is an eligible expense, the plan will reimburse these claims at 100%.

Most plans are written to include a family out of pocket maximum as well.

Please note that the allowed amount is critical to understanding what amounts may be applied to the plan deductible, what may be paid or even which portion is not covered.

I discuss allowed amounts in detail in Chapter 7 - Reimbursement.

COPAY

Most health insurance plans are written with the expectation that plan members will share in the cost of healthcare. A copay is one of these ways.

A copay is a fixed amount that a patient is required to pay for certain healthcare services, normally office visits. The copay is collected from the patient upfront and this copay amount cannot be billed to the health plan for reimbursement.

Copays can be tied to:

- Surgery
- Emergency room visits
- Urgent care visits
- Therapy visits
- DME
- Allergy tests
- X-rays
- Lab work

- Scans
- Inpatient care
- Prescriptions
- Office visit
- Mental health services
- Injections

The average copay is about $5.00 - $25.00 per office visit and $100.00 - $500.00 for other services like surgery and hospital admissions. The patient is required to pay the copay amount for each encounter.

Depending on how the plan is written, payment of the copay may be charged, even if the out of pocket maximum has been met in full. Some health plans are written to include a separate out of pocket maximum just for copays meaning once you have paid the stated amount, you will not have to pay another copay for the duration of the plan year.

In a nutshell

Copays are relatively small, upfront costs that are a requirement of some of the managed care plans, primarily HMO plans.

A copay is usually much cheaper than a plan deductible; the average plan deductible usually starts at around $100.00 and can reach several thousands of dollars.

For patients that only see a medical provider once or twice per year, and can afford it, a small copay is an excellent way to minimize their out of pocket costs while still giving them access to the care they need.

But for patients that visit a doctor frequently, say several visits per year, a $20.00 per visit copay that is payable each visit may pose a hardship. A patient may end up paying the equivalent of a low end deductible by the end of the year.

Perhaps one purpose of copays may be to try to make plan members mindful of the staggering cost of healthcare so they can try to control costs.

The thought is that, "if you have to pay for it, you will make sure you really need it."

For example, you may choose the lowest, least expensive level of care, you may opt to start with over-the-counter drugs as a way to treat minor ailments or injuries, you may schedule a visit with a medical provider and not use the emergency room to treat a cold or a small laceration and you may choose to limit the amount of doctors you see for a particular ailment.

Of course, the flip side to this is that copays are a deterrent for the plan members who just cannot afford them. Imagine a family of five needing to see a doctor but having to come up with a $20.00 copay, per person. This may mean that critical care could be delayed and a minor condition could end up costing way more than it should have because care was not sought early.

COINSURANCE

Most health insurance plans are written with the expectation that plan members will share in the cost of healthcare. Coinsurance is one of these ways.

The coinsurance amount is the percentage that the insurance carrier pays a claim at and the percentage that the patient is expected to pay, out of their pocket, toward the total claim.

One of the first questions the health carrier is asked when they are called to verify benefits and eligibility is, what is the coinsurance amount?

The coinsurance amount is usually the same for all services. But it is not unusual to see a plan that has a lower coinsurance amount for some therapies like occupational, physical, chiropractic, mental health or even for durable medical equipment and supplies. Also, the coinsurance percentage will differ greatly for in network vs. out of network services.

Let's look at the following example:

ABC PLAN:

$300.00 INDIVIDUAL DEDUCTIBLE
$900.00 FAMILY DEDUCTIBLE
$3000.00 MAX OUT OF POCKET
80% IN NETWORK
50% OUT OF NETWORK

In this case, ABC plan is expected to pay 80% of allowed charges, leaving the patient to pay the remaining 20% for in network providers. This plan also pays at 50% of allowed charges for out of network providers; leaving the patient to pay the remaining 50%.

So why is this important?

Revenue management is critical to the work that we do. We need to know what accounts have outstanding balances, why the balance is still due and what the possibility is for collection in full. We also need to collect every dime that is due from a patient, before they leave the office. Understanding the plan's coinsurance amounts is critical to collecting the right amount upfront.

Real world example

Medical Billers often bill claims for medical providers. But also, they may need to bill claims to help a patient get reimbursed, usually when services have been paid in full, upfront. Frequently, patients will call to complain about the low/no level of reimbursement that they received on a claim. Recently, a patient called me with such a complaint. Because I am in the "people business," I usually have them fax over the EOB to me for review.

Within two minutes I had figured out what had happened. Her claim was paid at 60% coinsurance instead of the 90% coinsurance amount that she was expecting. In fact, it took me longer to get ahold of the insurance company to fix it, than it did to find out the problem. The coinsurance amount is usually the first thing I focus on when I am reviewing EOB's for reimbursement.

Coinsurance amounts are fairly predictable. Low coinsurance amounts usually mean that the claim was paid out of network and the higher coinsurance amounts usually mean that the claim was paid in network. This may help you to quickly identify any claims that may not have been paid as expected.

Allowed amounts are critical to reimbursement. See the section on allowed amounts for a full explanation of how the allowed amount will impact claim payment.

I discuss allowed amounts in detail in Chapter 7- Reimbursement.

PARTICIPATING PROVIDER

Today, it is almost impossible to find a medical provider that does not participate with at least one health insurance carrier.

So what does this mean?

Most managed care plans are designed to deliver a two-tiered approach to the delivery of healthcare- in network and out of network.

In order for this concept to work it must:

- Have a large selection of participating providers (of all specialties, nationwide, small cities and large) for patients to choose from.
- Provide an incentive for a patient to want to use a participating provider.
- Provide an incentive for a provider to want to participate.
- Be delivered in way to control costs while still providing great care.

So it all starts with a network

Health insurance carriers are in the business of writing and administering health plans but they are also in the business of provider enrollment. A large, diverse, network of providers is critical to their ability to bring on new groups, keep customers satisfied and retain the business they have.

Providers must also provide great medical care to the patients that they treat. In order to afford to stay in business, they have to be open to the concept of plan participation because it helps to drive the constant flow of patients needed to stay in business and stay profitable.

Plan members in group plans usually will have no input into the plan that is ultimately selected for them. They will simply enroll, then figure out how to make that plan work for them. Provider selection is key. Plan members want to have access to medical providers, of all specialties, located in their neighborhood. They also want a huge network of medical providers to choose from so that the wonderful doctor they have had for years, that their family loves, is part of their plan network and they will not have to switch.

When a provider decides they want to participate in a health carrier's network, the process is fairly simple, they can contact the carrier online, click the ***provider enrollment*** button and get the process started.

As part of the process, the provider will agree, by signature, to ALL of the rules to participate; some of which include: *thou must provide quality care*, accept the plan allowed amounts, agree not to balance bill the patient over the allowed amounts and know how to handle claim disputes.

Once all of the paper work is completed, the provider is now a participating provider and their name will be listed in the provider directory. All plan members have access to the plan's provider directory, either online or hardcopy. This directory lists all providers, by area and specialty and is the go-to place when a plan member is trying to locate a medical provider.

In a nutshell

It is almost mandatory that a provider participate in at least one health plan since most plan members are enrolled under some type of managed care plan. This is the best way for a provider to ensure that a patient will find them when they need care.

It is not unusual for providers to participate with numerous, different health plans at the same time. Their names will be listed in the directories of all of these carriers. This ensures that they will have access to patients under a wide variety of health plans. A doctor can be participating with Aetna, Cigna and United Health care at the same time and will be able to treat patients who are insured with all of these plans.

It all comes down to expectations. A provider can expect lower reimbursement in exchange for access to more patients. A patient can expect higher reimbursement and less out of pocket costs. Lastly, a health carrier can expect some control over healthcare costs.

NON-PARTICIPATING PROVIDER

Providers that choose not to participate in a health insurance carrier's network of doctors are called non-participating or out of network providers.

Choosing to opt out of participation with a particular health carrier may not mean that a provider does not participate with any health plans. For example, a provider may be participating with Anthem but choose not to participate with Cigna. It is totally up to the provider to decide.

A provider may choose not to participate with a health carrier for a lot of reasons, including:

- Maybe the patient demographic just doesn't support the need to participate with a particular network. For example, the provider primarily treats Medicare patients of which they are participating, so they see no reason to add other networks.
- A provider may opt not to participate in a network despite the possibility of an influx of new patients because it may not be enough to offset the loss in income due to low contracted rates.
- The service provided has little competition. For example a durable medical supplier may have an item that is unique and necessary so that patients will contact them, whether in network or out. This was

the case a few years ago with the power scooters. Patients wanted one and they were willing to go out of network to buy one.

- The provider is currently out of network and they see no reason to change things.
- Non-participating providers have the option of billing the patient for any amounts not paid by the health plan. This means that they are assured that all billed claims will be paid in full. They are unwilling to reduce their profits by accepting the health carrier's allowed amounts.

To remain out of network is simple, they just don't enroll. Their name will not be listed in any of the provider directories. So how does a non-participating provider gain patients? Well, patient access could be based upon:

- Location of the provider, maybe they are part of a busy medical center.
- By referral from one provider to another.
- By patient word of mouth.
- By some form of advertising.

Since selection by provider directory is so random anyway, no one can really predict the number of patients that any provider may have access to using this method alone.

In a nutshell

The decision whether to participate in a network is totally up to the provider. Some providers may choose not to participate with a particular health carrier or may choose not to participate with any health carriers.

I think the jury is still out on whether the access to new plan members really does balance out the loss in income due to the low contracted rates.

It is assumed that choosing to remain out of network will affect a provider financially because patients are just not willing to pay the higher out of network costs; especially if there is a provider, in network, that can provide the same service. Also, some plans are written to provide no access to an out of network provider. This means that a patient will receive no reimbursement, at all, for any service performed by an out of network provider.

But we must not underestimate the draw of a good doctor. A physician who knows all aspects of your health, or who has been part of your family for years has a certain appeal that cannot be discredited. I know people who are willing to pay the higher out of pocket costs, just to keep their doctor. A good doctor who sees you as a person and not an ailment is a special quality, to some, and may be worth the extra costs associated with continuing being treated by them.

PRIMARY CARE PHYSICIAN

Managed care plans are written with a focus on delivering the best care while managing healthcare costs. A Primary Care Physician is another of the ways that a health insurance carrier will seek to control costs. A Primary Care Physician (PCP) can be thought of as a gate keeper in that they hold the keys to the kingdom; so to speak.

Real world example

A patient, new to an HMO plan, schedules a visit with his Primary Care Physician requesting a referral to a chiropractor for his back pain. He has had this problem off and on for years. It is usually no big deal, it flares up and after a few chiropractic visits, he is good as new. Because he has always had a PPO plan, he never had to get "permission" in the form of a referral before; he could just see any doctor he wanted to.

His Primary Care Physician requests a back x-ray. The patient knows this is not going to yield anything more than a soft tissue injury. The x-ray is negative for anything serious, so his Primary Care Physician diagnoses him with a soft tissue injury of some sort, writes him a prescription for muscle relaxants and pain pills, and tells him to come back in 4 weeks if it has not improved. No referral to a Chiropractor is given at this stage. It takes the patient two more trips before he can convince the PCP to issue the referral.

The role of the Primary Care Provider

This example, loosely, describes the Primary Care Provider's role. A PCP is tasked with deciding what medical services should be allowed, if a referral to a specialist is warranted and what is deemed necessary to treat the current condition. All services must be approved by the PCP.

The PCP will try to manage the level of care that each patient needs based on their current condition. The goal is to try to start with the lowest, most inexpensive level of care and move up to higher, more expensive and extensive, levels of care as needed.

Of course, any patient that exhibits any severe, life threating, serious or concerning injuries or illnesses will immediately be elevated to the highest level of care and reduced to lower levels of care as needed.

Keep in mind that most patients can be easily managed in a lower level of care. Colds, minor illnesses, some chronic or controlled conditions and even certain injuries may not require numerous visits, a specialist or admittance to a hospital. Their condition may easily be remedied with medication and time.

The PCP is tasked with understanding and treating a patient in the best possible way to ensure the overall wellbeing of the patient. But this does not mean that they are always right; all plans have a method to dispute or complain about the treatment or care that was received.

Managed care plans usually will have you select a Primary Care Provider upon enrollment and you will have the option to change this PCP if he leaves or if you become unsatisfied with the care that is provided.

ID CARD

Once a plan member enrolls with a health plan, they are provided with an Identification (ID) card. This card is critical to medical providers and billers as this small card provides tons of information about the plan.

Appearance

All identification cards are about the same size as a credit card but they are unique to the health carrier that issued them. They all provide the health carrier's name, and maybe the logo, and they all have distinctive card colors and formats. This way you can tell, at a glance, what health carrier the patient belongs too.

The Front of the ID Card

Every ID card issued by all of the different health carriers may be similar in look but the information provided could be totally different. Generally, on the front of the card you will find the group number, member name and ID number and on some ID cards you will also see the names of all dependents that are eligible under the plan.

You may also find the:

- Effective date of coverage

- Type of plan: PPO, HMO, FFS, POS etc.
- Copay amounts by type of service i.e. Office, Preventative, Specialty, Urgent care etc.
- Name and phone number of the Primary Care Physician
- Prescription numbers
- Deductibles
- Coinsurance amounts
- Dental and Vision information

The Back of the ID Card

Again, the information provided on the ID card could differ by health carrier but generally the back of the card is usually all about contact information, including:

- Phone numbers of member services, provider services, utilization review, the 24 helpline, etc.
- Insurance carrier name, address and phone numbers.
- Mailing address on where to bill claims.
- Numbers to call if you are admitted to a hospital or have a medical emergency.

Just FYI

The identification card is presented to the provider when a patient comes in the office, the provider should keep a copy of the front and the back of the ID card.

An identification card is not a guarantee of coverage or eligibility – the ID card is never confiscated when coverage ends so it is possible that a patient could give you a card and no longer have health insurance coverage.

Some health carriers will change the member ID number yet all other aspects of the card remain the same.

For this reason, some patients will not swap out the old card they are carrying for the new card. Using the old ID card could result in coverage and eligibility issues and claim denials. Calling the carrier to verify coverage is key.

The way a name is entered on the ID card should be the same way a claim is entered in the billing system and the same way the claim is billed to the health carrier. The name on the card is the name the health carrier has on file for this patient.

For Example

The patient's name is Elizabeth Smith, yet the patient prefers to go by Beth Smith. Because the billed claim will differ from the name in the health carrier's system, they may reject the claim.

In a Nutshell

The ID card provides some great information but it is not a substitute for calling the health carrier directly to confirm benefits and eligibility. The ID card is only part of what is needed to make sure that the visit will result in a paid claim.

SUMMARY PLAN DESCRIPTION

Upon enrollment in a health plan, the plan member is provided with a booklet that describes the benefits and limits of the plan. This booklet may be referred to by numerous different terms including a Certificate of Coverage, Benefit Booklet, Summary Plan Description, Health Plan Document or even a Policy.

This booklet is simply a guide to everything you ever wanted to know about a health plan; from what is covered and not covered to everything in between.

How is the Summary Plan Description Used?

Insurance carriers refer to this guide as a means to:

- Document the agreed upon terms and provisions of the plan.
- Understand and communicate the provisions of the plan.
- Adjudicate all claims in accordance with the provisions of the plan.

Patients will refer to this guide as a means to:

- Understand how they should access care.
- Determine how to enroll dependents.

- Understand their rights when employment is terminated.

Providers will refer to this guide as a means to:

- Understand the benefits and limits of the plan so that the patient can be advised, upfront, of any financial liability.
- Understand the rules of the plan.
- Make sure that the insurance carrier is administering the plan as written and that any gray areas can be clarified without penalty to the patient or the provider.

Billing Specialists will refer to this guide as a means to:

- Understand how to appeal all denied or incorrect payments.
- Challenge a provision or benefit that may not be administered as written or may be unclear.

From Experience...

Having spent over 30 years in this industry, I continue to use the SPD to help me when I need to draft an appeal letter that hits all of the high points, including:

- The basis for my appeal.
- The language in the SPD that supports my appeal.
- Any gray areas that can be interpreted either for or against the service I am trying to get approved. (Any ambiguity could work to a member's favor.)
- How the item I am trying to get approval for compares to other similar, but covered, items in the plan.

Referring to the SPD helps me to understand whether I even have a basis for appeal.

For Example:

A patient is having hearing problems and after having some hearing tests performed, they determine that a hearing aid is medically warranted for the patient. The SPD is consulted and they exclude all hearing services including hearing aids.

At this point, an appeal would not change the outcome since the plan clearly excludes coverage for hearing aids.

What information does the SPD contain?

A Summary Plan Description (SPD) provides pages and pages of detailed information about the plan, including:

- Benefits of the plan – deductible, out of pocket, etc.
- Provisions of the plan
- What is covered
- What is not covered
- How a particular service may be covered i.e., hospital, outpatient, office visit
- Plan limits
- Plan exclusions
- Requirements of the plans
- Who is covered
- How coverage begins and ends
- Cobra
- Grievance procedures
- ERISA

- Health carrier information
- Enrollment information
- Prescription coverage
- Coordination of Benefits
- Subrogation
- General provisions
- Definitions

CONSOLIDATED OMNIBUS BUDGET RECONCILIATION ACT

COBRA, the Consolidated Omnibus Budget Reconciliation Act of 1985, allows you to continue your health insurance in situations where coverage may have been lost due to certain qualifying events, i.e. the loss of employment (unless due to gross misconduct), divorce, death of a spouse or because a dependent child has reached the age of attainment. You are guaranteed the right to continue your existing group coverage provided that:

- Your employer has more than 20 employees.
- You were covered under the existing health plan.
- You have one of the qualifying events.
- You are able to pay the full cost of the premium yourself.

Costs

COBRA coverage is expensive since your employer will no longer be contributing toward the cost of your health insurance. Be prepared to pay 102% of the cost of the plan. The extra 2% is for administration fees. If you extend your COBRA coverage because of a disability, your premium will increase to 150% of cost.

Why Enroll in COBRA

Here are two very important reasons why, in spite of the cost, you may want to consider Cobra as a way to bridge the gap until you have other coverage:

1. The cost to treat even a minor illness or injury is very expensive. It is important that you always have some type of health insurance that can help offset the cost of needed care.
2. In order not to be subject to a preexisting period, one must not lose coverage for more than 63 days. COBRA allows you to bridge the period from when you lose coverage to when you enroll in a new plan.

Qualifying Events

- Termination of job or reduction in hours would entitle you and your eligible dependents to COBRA coverage for 18 months.
- Divorce, legal separation, death of the employee or if you are covered under Medicare would entitle your spouse and eligible dependents up to 36 months in COBRA coverage.
- Loss of dependent child status would entitle the child up to 36 months of COBRA coverage.
- Persons on disability and eligible for SSI would be entitled to COBRA coverage for up to 29 months.

Enrollment Time Line

- Your employer has 30 days to notify the plan holder of a qualifying event.
- The plan holder has 14 days to get your COBRA information and enrollment materials out to you.
- You or your dependents have 60 days to elect COBRA.
- You have 45 days to pay the first premium.

When Will Coverage Terminate?

- When you stop paying the premiums.
- If you move out of the coverage area.
- Your coverage period has run out.
- You become covered under another group plan.
- You become eligible for Medicare.

General Facts about COBRA

- Cobra is not available for individual plans; it applies to group plans only.
- Self-funded plans must also offer COBRA coverage.
- COBRA does not extend your life insurance.
- The employer, nor the insurance carrier, is required to send you monthly premium statements. It is up to you to get the correct cost of your premium in on time.
- If the employer is hit with a rate increase, your premiums can increase as well.
- Your COBRA coverage must be identical to the coverage you had before.
- You are allowed to drop incidental coverages like vision or dental plans.

UTILIZATION REVIEW

Managed care plans balance the need to provide plan members with access to good care, while at the same time utilizing different methods in an effort to control healthcare costs.

Utilization Review is one of these cost saving methods that most health plans rely on to help them manage and monitor the care that patients receive by directing patients to the appropriate levels of care. Depending on what care is needed, the Utilization Review Department (UR) will be the point of contact for all utilization review related inquiries.

The most common levels of Utilization Review are:

Prior Authorization – is the process of obtaining "permission," in advance, to have needed medical services performed. For example, a plan may require that prior authorization be obtained for all CT Scans. The patient's doctor would be required to contact the UR Department to request authorization and to provide the medical necessity to support the needed service. The UR Department will then provide the written authorization based on this need. **Failure to obtain a needed authorization, prior to the visit, could result in nonpayment of the claim.**

Pre-Certification - is the process of obtaining "permission," for a patient to be admitted to the hospital.

Some carriers also require pre-certification for certain out-patient surgical procedures and outpatient hospital stays.

The back of the patient's ID card will provide the telephone number of where to call in the event that pre-certification is needed. The doctor, the hospital, even the patient or his family can call to start the pre-certification process. Do keep in mind, the patient, or his family, may not be able to complete the process as they may lack the required medical information such as: diagnoses, appropriate codes, anticipated length of stay, etc.

Normally, pre certification is handled in advance, but in the case of emergencies you may have a reasonable amount of time, up to 24 to 36 hours, in which to pre-certify. **Failure to pre-certify could result in the reduction or denial of benefits.**

Pre-determination- is the process of requesting prior approval for a proposed surgery or service. A pre-determination letter is basically a letter that details the type of service, approximate costs, attending physician, hospital information, patient history, any supporting test results and/or clinical information that will support the medical necessity for the needed surgery or service.

It is good idea to request pre-determination for cases where a very expensive, unique or specialty service/surgery is to be performed. This is a way to find out, in advance, if the procedure would be covered under the plan. **Pre-determination normally takes about 30 days for a final decision to be rendered.**

Concurrent Review- is a request for care at the same time that treatment is being rendered. For example, a patient that is hospital confined for a long period of time may be followed by the UR Department, every week or so, just to monitor the care and/or suggests ways to control cost, etc.

Retrospective Review- is a request for care after the service is rendered.

REFERRAL

Managed care plans are designed to provide plan members access to the care they need but at the same time they also need to control health care costs. This is accomplished, in part, by making sure that some front end controls are in place. One such control is the Referral.

Some types of managed care plans do not allow a patient to see any provider they choose to (unless they are willing to pay for the visit in full) without a referral on file.

Let's say that a plan member has noticed that her hearing has started to decline in her right ear. She decides to see a doctor and discovers that there is an Ear, Nose and Throat doctor located in the medical center just down the street.

If she has an HMO plan, she may not have access to this ENT doctor, ever, unless she is granted a referral or the doctor is in network. Without a valid referral she must be willing to pay for the visit and all subsequent follow up care, in full; with no chance of being reimbursed by her health plan.

If she has a PPO, she could have some coverage from an out of network provider.

What is a referral?

Depending on the rules of the managed care plan, some patients that are in need of specialty care, whether it be care that is not available in the current network or simply a wish to see that new doctor down the street, must first obtain written permission from their Primary Care Physician.

This permission slip is called a referral.

A referral provides written authorization for patients to obtain services or specialty care that either cannot be provided by the Primary Care Physician or cannot be provided in network. **Seeking a referral based on a desire to see any doctor of their choice is usually not approved.**

The PCP's office is responsible for determining, in advance, if the request is warranted; based on medical necessity. If approved, the PCP will provide a copy for the patient to take with them to their initial visit with the out-of-network provider or specialist.

So how does a referral control health care cost?

Providers that enroll with managed care plans agree to accept the allowed amount that the health carrier deems appropriate and not balance bill the patient for the difference. Since the health carrier is not going to pay the claim at the amount the provider would normally bill, which is usually much higher than the allowed amount, the plan is saving money.

Primary care doctors usually refer patients only to contracted providers, this way the provider can expect to be paid at the allowed amount and the health carrier is saving money.

Primary Care doctors are tasked with making sure that the level of care fits the condition. Meaning you will not be referred to a surgeon with a complaint of arm pain. The Primary Care doctor will manage your care with conservative treatment first, i.e. x-rays, splints, prescriptions, etc., and if no improvement has been made you will move to the next level of care. Monitoring and directing the level of care needed based on condition, saves money.

In a nutshell

Under some plans, a Referral is mandatory. Failure to obtain a needed referral, prior to the visit, could result in nonpayment of the claim.

ELIGIBILITY

For all new patients, the first thought should always be of eligibility:

- Is the patient eligible under the plan?
- Is the service eligible for coverage under the plan?
- Who is eligible for coverage under the health plan?

Is the patient eligible under the plan is fairly simple to confirm. You simply must call the health carrier directly or visit them online. Just because a patient has an ID card, does not mean they are currently still eligible for coverage.

If checking eligibility online, you will receive pages and pages of data. Take the time to thoroughly review all pages of the inquiry. You may learn that the plan provides less coverage than what may have appeared at first glance.

Is the service eligible for coverage under the plan is also fairly easy to confirm. You can call the health carrier to obtain coverage information by phone or by fax. You can also review a copy of the patient's plan booklet or Summary Plan Description (SPD). The question should not only be, is the service eligible for coverage? But also…

- Do I or the patient fit the current parameters for coverage?
- Does the service have to be performed in a particular setting to be eligible for coverage? For example, a hospital instead of a provider's office.
- Does the patient have to be a certain age to be eligible? It is not unusual, especially with some state Medicaid plans, that coverage for certain services be available only to plan members under a certain age. For example, children under the age 21 may have coverage for vision while vision services are totally excluded for all adults.
- Does the patient's current condition fit the criteria for coverage? Most health carriers have a list of medical coverage policies on various procedures, surgeries and supplies. These coverage policies provide the criteria in which a particular service, supply or treatment, will be covered.

For example, let's look at Dermabrasion, Chemical Peels.

Dermabrasion, Chemical Peels is covered under most health plans, provided the criteria for coverage is met. The Medical Coverage Policy may state that:

Coverage for Dermabrasion, Chemical Peels will be forthcoming for the diagnosis of Actinic Keratosis (precancerous skin lesions) but coverage will be denied for the treatment of wrinkles or a tattoo removal.

The criteria may also go further and require that a certain number of lesions be present and that other treatments, medications or therapies be tried first. Medical Coverage Policies can be found online at the health carrier's website.

Who is eligible for coverage under the health plan can be a little more tricky. Just because someone is a family member does not make them eligible for coverage. For example, in spite of the fact that a lot of grandparents are raising their grandchildren, they may not be eligible for coverage under a plan until they are formally adopted.

The people that are normally eligible for coverage include:

Spouse- Your legal spouse. Coverage for the spouse will cease once a divorce is final. If COBRA is available, the ex-spouse would be able to apply for continued coverage under the COBRA plan.

Dependent children- Unmarried children that are under the age of attainment. This normally includes natural, stepchildren and children placed under the legal guardianship of the employee.

Newborns- State law requires that newborns be covered for the first 31 days of life. During this 31-day period, the child must be added to the plan and any applicable premiums must be paid. Dependents not added within the 31-day period might be subject to additional underwriting.

Adopted children- Normally, adopted children can be added to the plan as soon as the employee takes custody of the child- pending the final adoption.

Common Law Marriage- Typically, this refers to a "marriage' without the benefit of a legal ceremony. Unless the plan recognizes common law marriages or the plan includes coverage for domestic partners, the partner would not qualify as an eligible dependent under the health plan and therefore cannot be covered.

Physically handicapped, dependent children- You can extend coverage for physically handicapped children beyond the age of 26; depending on the disability.

SUBROGATION

Most health insurance plans include a Subrogation Clause that allows them to recover any money that was paid toward healthcare expenses that resulted from injuries or an illness that were caused by a negligent third party.

Such examples could be related to an auto accident, injury on someone's property, malpractice, product defect, dog bite, slip and fall or any other type of injury where a third party is deemed to be liable.

An example of how subrogation would work

You are involved in an auto accident, caused by the other driver, and you receive substantial injuries that render you unable to work while you recover.

Because of your injuries, you incur bills from numerous different medical providers and facilities; from hospital and ambulance charges to lab and imaging services to physical therapy and medical supplies. All of these claims are billed to and paid for by your health insurance carrier.

Since your injuries are due to no fault of your own, you file suit against the negligent third party in an attempt to be compensated for your pain, suffering, lost wages, etc.

Your case is finally settled and your health insurance carrier, based on the Subrogation Clause, is entitled to be reimbursed for all, or a portion, of what they paid out for the accident related medical expenses that were incurred. Most attorneys will build this into the settlement.

So how does your health carrier know that your care was due to a negligent third party?

In a lot of cases, especially for severe injuries, it is evident that an accident has occurred and the hospital, ambulance and medical records will fully support this.

But what if the accident only resulted in relatively minor injuries?

The health carrier will still subrogate. If the health carrier suspects that your condition may be related to an accident of any kind, they will ask you at the time of treatment to provide detail on how the injury occurred. They may also send you a letter asking you again about the injury.

Real world example

I decided to join this "get fit" challenge and during the course of doing more than I should have, I hurt my knee. By the next morning my knee was swollen so I decided to have it looked at by my doctor. He asked and I explained how it happened. After giving me the side eye and telling me that walking - at my age- would be much more beneficial, I was released with only a minor soft tissue injury.

About two weeks later, I received a letter in the mail from my health carrier asking, again, how the injury occurred in detail and by signature I acknowledged that ***the information given herein is true and correct*** and that ***I authorize my plan to verify any information contained in the document.*** Make no mistake, your health insurance carrier will ask, and if not satisfied, they will pursue it.

You might ask why not just bill the third party up-front for all related claims?

The reason why this does not usually happen is because it may take years for a case to be investigated, litigated and the proceeds disbursed. It would be unreasonable for providers to wait for payment while the case is settled.

Besides, you want to have full access to the providers that can help get you well without having to worry about large overdue bills.

LETTER OF AGREEMENT

A letter of agreement is a signed contract between the provider of service and the health carrier in which they agree to the terms for how a particular claim or series of claims will be reimbursed.

The health carrier, or the provider, may try to initiate a Letter of Agreement based on the needs of a patient. This is a legal, binding agreement that clearly spells out how each party should behave and what each side expects to happen.

A Letter of Agreement is usually signed by someone in authority. Usually someone that is capable of making that type of decision on behalf of the provider and the health carrier.

Health carriers may use a Letter of Agreement as a way to:

1. Negotiate a reimbursement rate for a particular service, treatment or supply.

For example: A durable medical supply may have an invoice cost of $300.00 but the health carrier may try to negotiate with the provider of service to bring that price down to $255.00 in exchange for an agreement to pay the claim within 12 business days.

2. Lessen a patient's liability.

For example: The durable medical supplier agrees to accept the $255.00 for the item with the understanding that they also must agree not to bill the patient the difference between the $300.00 invoice and the negotiated price of $255.00.

A provider of service may use a Letter of Agreement as a means to:

1. Gain access to a patient that may be out of network but is in need of the service that the provider can provide.

For Example: A patient may be in need of a unique prosthetic device, but the manufacturer is out of network. The health carrier and the provider can work together to allow the patient access to the needed item at a cost that may be below invoice cost.

2. Ensure correct and accurate payment for a service, treatment or supply that may be manually priced; (no current rate is on file for the service). The health carrier would then attempt to configure the cost. Usually this occurs most often for items that do not have a valid CPT-4/HCPCS code.

Health carriers usually have difficulty trying to price a service, supply or treatment that don't have a valid billing code. Negotiating this, in advance, is a way to ensure fair reimbursement and prompt payment.

GAP EXCEPTION

A GAP exception is a written request to secure permission for services to be provided by an out of network provider. The out of network provider will be reimbursed the same way as if an in network provider performed the service.

Managed care plans are written to restrict access to out of network providers. The hope is that the health carrier's provider network includes hundreds of different providers, of all specialties, in all areas, so the need to go out of network would be minimal.

A network of providers that are able to provide every type of service that a patient may need is not always possible. Access to some services, especially unique services like prosthetic and orthotics, durable medical equipment, therapy and others, may not be possible without a GAP exception because most patients are unable to afford the high out of pocket costs associated with going out of network.

A GAP exception is exactly as it sounds, it bridges that gap where no in network coverage exists by providing a bridge to an out of network provider.

A provider may initiate the GAP exception by formally asking the health carrier to approve the out of network service. The health carrier will ask for all documentation that supports the need for the service and they will make sure that they have no one in network that can perform the same service.

Most health plans understand that GAP exceptions are part of providing great care to their plan members. It is not a patient's fault when the network fails to have adequate in network coverage. As long as medical necessity can be supported, approval for care is normally granted.

Once approved, the patient will have access to the out of network provider without having to worry about the high out of network costs since the service would be paid as if in network.

MEDICAL NECESSITY

Every health plan that is issued by a health insurance carrier, whether it's a commercial health carrier, Medicare or Medicaid, is built on the premise that every treatment, service or supply must be medically necessary. Medical necessity simply means that all care must have a medical reason or a medical need to be performed.

Trying to rule out a particular condition, hoping to ease a patient's fears or perhaps, just wanting to have a certain service, treatment or supply does not make it medically necessary.

For Example

You go to see a doctor with the vague complaint of chest pain. Chest pain could be from multiple sources, i.e. heart, muscle, soft tissue, upper abdomen, upper back or various other locations. That is why a doctor will try to isolate the pain asking specific questions, including:

- When does it occur?
- Where is it located?
- What is the severity?
- How long have you had it?

Usually by the end of the inquiry, they will have some general idea what the problem may be and they will order the appropriate medically necessary tests in the hope of confirming a diagnosis so that treatment can begin. All appropriate tests would be considered medically necessary.

In treating this same patient with the complaint of chest pain, let's say that a doctor decides to perform an x-ray of the foot. That x-ray may not be considered medically necessary unless the doctor can make a clear connection between the chest pain and the need to x-ray the foot.

Every Summary Plan Description or plan booklet contains a clear definition of medical necessity and most read about the same. When in doubt refer to the plan for clarity.

CHAPTER THREE TEST

Directions: Using what you have learned in Chapter Three, answer the following questions.

1. What does timing have to do with the plan deductible?
2. Why do plans have a family deductible?
3. What does the term out of pocket mean?
4. Copay and coinsurance are considered two forms of what?
5. Why would a provider choose to participate in a network?
6. Why would a provider choose not to participate in a network?
7. What is the role of a PCP?
8. A patient has an ID card does that mean they have health coverage?
9. What is the role of Utilization Review?
10. What may be the most compelling reason to take COBRA in spite of the cost?
11. Who would a referral most likely be issued for a patient to have access to?
12. GAP Exceptions and Letters of Agreements are requested for what reason?
13. True or False. Being ordered/requested by a medical provider meets the standard of medically necessary.

4 CODING

Chapter Overview - There are so many different types of medical codes and all of them are critical- with no room for error. In this chapter, we will look at the various forms of coding.

This Chapter Includes:

BILLING VS. CODING

What is medical coding and billing?

Coding is a term that is used to describe the process of selecting the appropriate code that accurately describes the patient's condition and the type of care that was provided. Correct coding generates from the provider's documentation of the encounter which is later translated into codes. Medical providers are responsible for assigning the correct ICD-10, CPT-4 and HCPCS codes, although they may use the assistance of a Procedural Coder to help.

Care must be taken to ensure that the right codes have been selected. Each code should be a perfect fit; this means it should not only perfectly describe the service or supply that was provided but also the patient's condition as well. If not a perfect fit, a miscellaneous code should be used with a special report attached that provides a more accurate and detailed description of the encounter.

Improper coding, whether it's accidental, intentional or due to lack of experience, could result in the doctor being "suspected" of fraud by the carrier. A provider could be subject to a fraud investigation beginning with an audit of his practice. If evidence of improper coding is found, the provider could face possible criminal and financial penalties and sanctions.

Billing is the process of taking those codes that were assigned by the provider, along with any particulars of the visit, including the patient and plan information and date of service, to complete a CMS 1500 claim form and bill the carrier for payment.

Medical Billers do not normally assign the codes that are billed. The pre-coded "trip slip" provides most of the codes needed to bill the claim correctly.

Care must be taken to ensure that a claim is billed correctly. Undocumented or unperformed services, exaggerating the complexity of the visit, changing dates to reflect eligible periods or changing the diagnosis to take advantage of plan benefits are all examples of fraud. Committing fraud sets the provider's practice, as well as, the Medical Biller up for potentially serious legal problems.

Although billers do not assign codes, they do have the responsibility of making sure that the claims that they bill all match up. This means that a biller should not ignore any claim that appears suspect. The codes should match the treatment and diagnosis, the dates and place of service must be accurate and the patient information should be correct.

A medical biller is expected to bill the claim based on the information that was provided on the coded trip slip but they also have the responsibility of making sure that the claim has everything it needs to meet the clean claim standard. The claim may require additional data or additional codes may be needed to ensure correct payment. A modifier, for example, may not be listed on the trip slip but it may be critical to ensuring correct reimbursement and is usually medical biller assigned.

Simply put, the medical billing process is all about taking great care to make sure that the claims that ***you*** bill are always of the highest quality and integrity, always accurate and always correct.

CPT-4 CODES

When we think of medical billing and coding, our first thought is of the coding systems that are critical to the process.

So what is a CPT-4 code anyway?

Current Procedural Terminology-4 (CPT-4) is the coding system that is used to provide a written description of the medical, surgical and diagnostic services that can be provided to a patient. CPT-4 codes are developed and maintained by the American Medical Association (AMA) and are updated yearly.

How are CPT-4 codes used?

A patient goes to the doctor complaining of being dizzy and having a headache. The doctor performs a new patient, problem focused exam and discovers that his blood pressure is elevated. He does a CT scan of the head and performs some blood work. All of his diagnostic tests are negative. The patient is diagnosed with high blood pressure and released home with medication.

CPT-4 codes allow the biller to describe every service and test that was provided to the patient in a concise and easy to understand format. Every service that a provider performs is translated from its word format into a CPT-4 code.

For example, a CT scan of the head is CPT-4 code 70470 (CT head w/wo contrast) and a new patient, problem focused exam is CPT-4 99201. Both of these codes, as well as the codes for the blood work, would be entered on the CMS 1500 form and billed to the carrier.

These codes tell the health insurance carrier everything about the patient's encounter. So even though they were not present at the date of service, they are able to determine exactly what occurred solely by the codes entered on the billed claim.

This starts with careful, detailed documentation of every aspect of the patient's visit, including: all of the services that were performed, what body part was involved, the detail or complexity of the visit- everything. This documentation is what will be used to determine which of the hundreds of CPT-4 codes are appropriate to use.

But CPT-4 coding is not as simple as picking a code that matches the service.

CPT-4 guidelines are strict and must be adhered to. Not every service can be billed, certain procedures are considered a normal part of the service, some services cannot be billed together, while other services, like multiple services same site, or same service different site, must be handled in accordance with the guidelines in the CPT-4 manual. The CPT-4 manual even lists guidelines on how office visits must be billed.

Coding is not a simple process, ALL of the rules must be adhered to or the provider's practice, and the biller, could be subject to unwanted scrutiny by the health carrier.

All of the rules are provided in the CPT-4 manual but you can also expand your knowledge by taking one of the Certified Procedural Coding classes and testing to obtain your Procedural Coding Certification.

CPT-4 codes are entered in field 24D of the CMS 1500 claim form.

CPT-4 Codes fall into three categories:

- Category I codes are procedure and service codes
- Category II codes are used for tracking and measurement.
- Category III codes are for new and developing technology, procedures, and services.

Code Sections

- Evaluation and Management
- Anesthesia
- Surgery
- Radiology
- Pathology and Laboratory Procedures
- Medicine Services and Procedures
- CPT-4 Modifiers

ICD-9 CODES

ICD-9 codes will no longer be used unless you are billing a claim that incurred prior to 10/1/15. But because these codes are so critical to the history of coding, no insurance manual will be complete without at least some mention of them.

So what is an ICD-9 code anyway?

ICD-9, International Classification of Diseases - Ninth Revision, is the coding system that is used to provide a written description of a patient's disease, illness, injury, symptoms or complaints which is then translated from its word format into an ICD-9 code. The ICD-9 booklet was updated by the AMA (American Medical Association) on a yearly basis.

ICD-9 codes are three digit, four digit and five digit codes that are listed in the ICD- 9 manual with code sets that range from 001.0 through V82.9. ICD-9 codes are required on all claims with a date of service prior to 10/1/15.

These codes tell the health insurance carrier everything about the patient's encounter. So even though they were not present when the patient was seen, they are able to determine exactly why the patient was being treated.

This starts with careful, detailed documentation of every aspect of the patient's reason for the visit:

- The patient's complaints.
- When the complaints started.
- Duration
- Severity
- What they were doing when it occurred.
- If they had it before.

This documentation is what will be used to determine which of the hundreds of ICD-9 codes are appropriate to use. **ICD-9 codes are entered in field 21 of the CMS 1500 claim form.**

ICD-9 codes are broken down in the following way:

3 digits represent the category:

- 250 - Diabetes

4 digits represent the subcategory:

- 250.1 Diabetes with ketoacidosis

5 digits represent the sub-classification:

- 250.13 Diabetes with ketoacidosis, type I [juvenile type], uncontrolled

Claims should always be coded to the highest level of specificity. This means that a 3 digit code should be used only if no valid 4 digit code is available. A four digit code should be used only if no valid 5 digit is available. If a valid 5 digit is available, it should always be used. Each additional digit within the code tells you more about the condition.

Why the change from ICD-9 to ICD-10?

- The new codes are alpha numeric codes.
- The code changed from five positions to seven.
- 13,000 codes under ICD-9 to 68,000 codes under ICD-10.
- ICD-10 has been expanded to fully describe the condition/disease/injury.
- Codes were added to reflect which side of the body.
- Codes were added to reflect the patient's trimester of pregnancy.
- It expanded the system so we would not run out of codes.
- The new codes would allow for more in depth review of disease and treatments to improve the outcomes.

The impact of changing from ICD-9 to 10 codes continues to be felt. Providers are complaining about the complexity of the new codes and a lot of providers continue to use the 'crosswalk,' which basically takes the old ICD-9 code and points them toward the exact same ICD-10 match.

The goal of the new ICD-10 codes was not to replace the old with a new look alike code. It was changed to obtain a clearer more precise diagnosis. Given a chance, the ICD-10 codes will provide a lot more data that will help us key into better ways to track outcomes and treat patients.

ICD-10 CODES

When we think of medical billing and coding, our first thought is of the coding systems that are critical to the process.

So what is an ICD-10 code anyway?

ICD-10, International Classification of Diseases- tenth revision, is used to report all healthcare diagnoses and conditions. Every disease/condition is translated from the word format into an ICD-10 code. This code is required when billing a claim as a way to report the patient's disease, illness, injury, symptoms, and complaints. The ICD-10 is copyrighted by the World Health Organization (WHO) and the ICD-10 manual is updated yearly.

How are ICD-10 codes used?

ICD-10 codes are designed to provide a fuller understanding of all aspects of a patient's condition.

For Example

Let's look at a diagnosis as simple as an allergic reaction; ICD-10 code T78.40. Depending on the specific condition, you could use the following ICD-10 codes:

- Pollen - code J30.1
- Peanuts - code Z91.010
- Seafood - code Z91.013
- Ragweed - code J30.0
- Drugs -code T78.40

These codes would further be expanded to provide specifics on the type of drug, what type of seafood, chronic or acute conditions, left or right, etc. As you can see, picking a code requires a higher level of information about the patient's condition; including how it occurred and what the patient was doing when it occurred.

These codes tell the health insurance carrier everything about the patient's encounter. So even though they were not present when the patient was seen, they are able to determine exactly why the patient was being treated.

This starts with careful, detailed documentation of every aspect of the patient's reason for the visit:

- The patient's complaints.
- When they started.
- Duration.
- Severity.
- What they were doing when it occurred.
- If they've had it before.

This documentation is what will be used to determine which of the hundreds of ICD-10 codes are appropriate to use. **ICD-10 codes are entered in field 21 of the CMS 1500 claim form.**

ICD-10 is New

Prior to 10/1/2015, the coding system in place was ICD-9. So what has changed?

- The new codes are alpha numeric codes.
- The code changed from five positions to seven.
- 13,000 codes under ICD-9 to 68,000 codes under ICD-10.
- ICD-10 has been expanded to fully describe the condition/disease/injury.
- Codes were added to reflect which side of the body.
- Codes were added to reflect the patient's trimester of pregnancy.
- It expanded the system so we would not run out of codes.

The new codes would allow for a more in depth review of a disease and its treatments in order to improve the outcomes.

Comparison of the new vs old codes

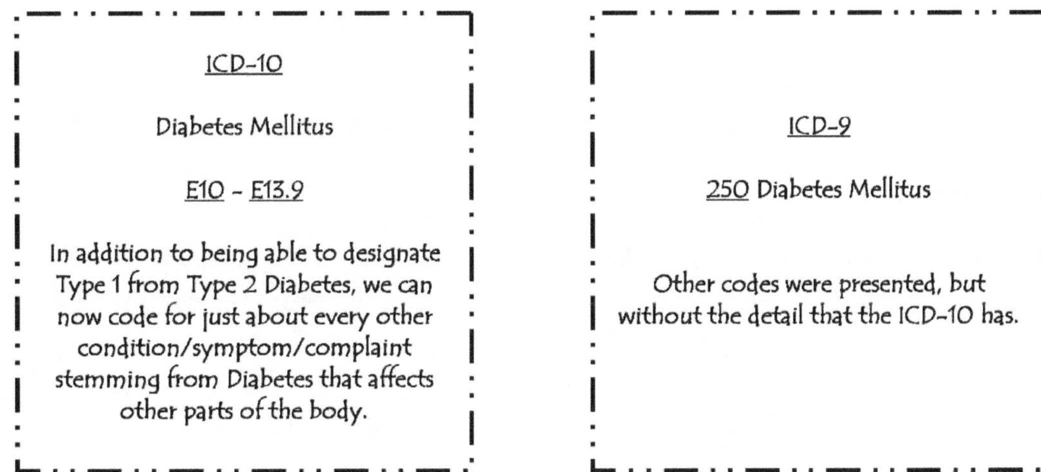

ICD-10 is the coding system in place effective 10/1/15

HCPCS CODES

When we think of medical billing and coding our first thought is of the coding systems that are critical to the process.

So what is a HCPCS Code?

A HCPCS (pronounced like hicks picks) code is not unlike any other billing code that is used to describe the service, treatment or supplies that can be provided to a patient. The unique difference is that these codes are divided into Level I and Level II codes.

- Level I HCPCS codes are five-digit numeric codes that look identical to and are used the same way as CPT-4 codes.
- Level II HCPCS codes are five-digit, alpha-numeric codes that are used to bill for non-physician services.

HCPCS II codes include, but are not limited to:

- Ambulance rides.
- Durable medical equipment.

- Alcohol and Drug abuse treatment.
- Miscellaneous Medical Services.
- Prosthetic and Orthotics.
- Medical supplies.
- Chemotherapy drugs.

HCPCS Level I

So why do we need both HCPCS Level I and CPT- 4 codes if they are identical?

This is a bit confusing but CPT-4 codes were designed for billing to private and commercial health insurance carriers and HCPCS level I codes were designed for billing to Medicare, Medicaid and some other payers. CMS adopted the same codes as the CPT-4, so for billing purposes the codes are the same but the main difference depends on who you are billing to.

For example

When 99214 is billed to a commercial carrier it is considered a CPT-4 code

and

When 99214 is billed to Medicare it is considered a HCPCS Level I code.

HCPCS Level II codes

HCPCS Level II codes are used to identify products, services, drugs and supplies, including durable medical equipment and they are used as temporary codes when a valid code does not exist yet.

PROVIDER NUMBERS

Although patients will identify providers by their given name, the way that a medical provider is identified by a health insurance carrier, and even the state they practice in, will be by one of the various provider numbers that will be assigned to them.

A medical provider is assigned numerous different provider numbers by their state, government as well as insurance carriers.

Examples:

1. The state assigns each new doctor a license number as proof that he passed all of the necessary requirements to practice medicine in the state where the license was issued.
2. A commercial insurance carrier will assign all new participating providers a unique provider number.
3. A new doctor will also be assigned a Tax ID number. This number is used to identify the provider of service and is also used for tax reporting.
4. CMS now assigns each doctor an NPI number, replacing the old UPIN number.
5. Durable medical suppliers may be assigned a taxonomy number.

Out of all of these numbers, the NPI number is most critical to billing. This number is required on every claim that is billed.

The Centers for Medicare and Medicaid Services (CMS) began issuing NPI numbers in 2007 as part of HIPAA. HIPAA's primary role is to protect patient information and to simplify and standardize the health insurance process.

The NPI number:

1. Identifies who is billing a claim.
2. Helps providers identify each other.
3. Helps clearinghouses standardize the way they create and transmit data.
4. Helps to identify who the treating provider is with regard to in-patient medical records.

This unique 10 digit number is used by all provider types and is permanent. Some of the providers that are required to have an NPI number include:

- Midwives
- Nurse Practitioners
- Dentists
- Chiropractors
- Pharmacy Technicians
- Doctors
- Physician's Assistants
- Hospitals
- Medical Device Companies
- Physical and Occupational Therapists

- Nursing Homes
- Laboratories

Depending on the health carrier's specific requirements, the NPI number may be used on some or all of these various places on the CMS 1500 form, including:

- 17B requiring a referring provider NPI number.
- 24J requiring a rendering provider NPI number.
- 32A and/or B requiring a service facility location NPI number.
- 33A and/or B requiring a billing provider's name, address and NPI number.

Providers are required to have and use this number when billing, even if they use an outside billing agency to bill claims. A medical biller is not required to have a NPI number. The NPI number of the provider that rendered the service will always be used instead.

Not only is this number critical to the billing process, it is also the number that you will be asked to provide when you call the carrier to verify benefits, eligibility or to check patient status.

The NPI number is also the number that is on all correspondence from the health plan; from checks and EOB's to requests for additional information and claim denials.

PLACE OF SERVICE CODES

A place of service code is a code used to tell where the service was performed. This code is mandatory and is entered on 24B of the CMS 1500 form.

The following is a list of the most common place of service codes. You can find the full list at www.cms.gov.

11	Office-Location, other than a hospital, Skilled Nursing Facility (SNF), Military Treatment Facility, Community Health Center, State or Local Public Health Clinic or Intermediate Care Facility (ICF), where the health professional routinely provides health examinations, diagnosis and treatment of illness or injury on an ambulatory basis.
12	Patient's Home-Location, other than a hospital or other facility, where the patient receives care in a private residence.
21	Inpatient Hospital-A facility, other than psychiatric, which primarily provides diagnostic, therapeutic (both surgical and nonsurgical) and rehabilitation services by, or under, the supervision of physicians to patients admitted for a variety of medical conditions.
22	Outpatient Hospital-A portion of a *hospital which provides diagnostic, therapeutic (both surgical and non-surgical), and rehabilitation services to sick or injured persons who do not require hospitalization or institutionalization.*
23	Emergency Room Hospital-A portion of a hospital where emergency diagnosis and treatment of illness or injury is provided.
24	Ambulatory Surgical Center-A freestanding facility, other than a physician's office, where surgical and diagnostic services are provided on an ambulatory basis.
25	Birthing Center-A facility, other than a hospital's maternity facilities or a physician's office, which provides a setting for labor, delivery and immediate postpartum care as well as immediate care of newborn infants.
26	Military Treatment Facility-A medical facility operated by one or more of the Uniformed Services. Military Treatment Facility (MTF) also refers to certain former U.S. Public Health Service (USPHS) facilities now designated as Uniformed Service Treatment Facilities (USTF).
31	Skilled Nursing Facility-A facility which primarily provides inpatient skilled nursing care and related services to patients who require medical, nursing, or rehabilitative services but does not provide the level of care or treatment available in a hospital.
32	Nursing Facility-A facility which primarily provides skilled nursing care and related services to residents for the rehabilitation of injured, disabled, or sick persons, or on a regular basis, health-related care services above the level of custodial care to other than mentally retarded individuals.
33	Custodial Care Facility-A facility which provides room, board, and other personal assistance services, generally on a long-term basis, and which does not include a medical component.
34	Hospice-A facility, other than a patient's home, in which palliative and supportive care for terminally ill patients and their families are provided.
41	Ambulance-Land-A land vehicle specifically designed, equipped, and staffed for lifesaving and transporting the sick or injured.
42	Ambulance-Air or Water-An air or water vehicle specifically designed, equipped, and staffed for lifesaving and transporting the sick or injured.
50	Federally Qualified Health Center-A facility located in a medically underserved area that provides Medicare beneficiaries

MODIFIERS

The completed CMS 1500 claim form is designed to tell a story about the patient's visit. The form can tell you who the patient is, what was wrong with them, what services were performed, when they were seen, and who treated them.

The goal of billing is to provide everything about that encounter so that the claim processor will have everything they need to accurately process the claim; at first pass. This means the usual information, including date of service, type and provider of service as well as any special circumstances, complex treatments or surgical support that was needed.

Since the CMS 1500 claim form is concise with very strict entry requirements and limited areas for documentation, a modifier is often used to further describe the events of the visit. A modifier is a two-digit code that is added to field 24D of the CMS 1500 form in order to alter, clarify or add to what has been reported on other areas of the claim.

Maybe the procedure that was being performed was so complex that it required more than one physician (modifier 62). Maybe the procedure was performed on a newborn weighing 2 pounds (modifier 63). Maybe the same procedure was performed on both sides (modifier 50 or LT and RT). Or maybe multiple procedures were performed during the same session (modifier 51).

Modifiers are a critical part of the billing process. Not only do they serve to provide clarity and detail but they also ensure that a claim will be paid correctly. If a modifier is incorrect or absent, it could result in a claim paying less than expected.

For Example

A patient is in need of physical therapy due to pain in her wrist. She obtains a referral from the primary care physician and preapproval from the health carrier. Therapy is rendered and the claim is billed to the health carrier. The claim is later denied because it lacked the information needed to complete processing. After a call to the health carrier, the biller discovers that the plan requires a modifier to indicate whether it was the left wrist (LT) or the right wrist (RT). The claim is corrected, rebilled and subsequently paid by the plan.

The CPT-4 manual provides the full list of modifiers, all designed to fit a wide range of different needs and situations. This should be your first stop when referencing modifiers and how they should be used.

Keep in mind that every situation is different and the rules for every health carrier may be different. One carrier may have mandatory requirements for certain modifiers while another carrier may consider that same modifier to be optional. Call the carrier or check their website online if you have questions about how a modifier should be used or if a modifier is appropriate for the claim that you are billing.

It bears repeating, using modifiers to distort the true complexity of the visit as a means to increase reimbursement may subject the provider's billing practice, and the biller, to unwanted scrutiny and incorrect reimbursement.

Refer to the 2016 CPT Manual for the full list (with descriptions) and the proper usage of all modifiers.

CHAPTER FOUR TEST

Directions: Using what you have learned in Chapter Four, answer the following questions.

1. What is the difference between coding and billing?

2. If a valid CPT-4 code does not exist, how should that claim be billed?

3. What is the difference between an ICD-10 code and a CPT-4 code?

4. Where would you find the rules and guidelines for appropriate use of CPT-4 codes?

5. The date of service is 9/1/15 but the claim is not billed until 1/5/16 should a ICD-9 or ICD-10 code be used?

6. What is the difference between HCPCS I and HCPCS II codes?

7. Out of all of the numbers that are assigned to a provider which one is the most often used?

8. What field on the CMS 1500 form does the Place of Service code go?

9. What is the purpose of a modifier?

10. Coding to the highest level of specificity means what?

5 BILLING

Chapter Overview - What is a clean claim? This chapter is all about the standard of clean claim and what you need to do to meet this standard every time; every claim.

This Chapter Includes:

Clean Claim

Assignment of Benefits

Clearinghouse

Electronic vs. Paper Claims

What You Need From The Patient

What Every Claim Needs

Coordination of Benefits

Timely Filing

CLEAN CLAIM

Clean claim refers to the process of making sure that a claim has everything needed for it to be processed at first submission. **That should be the goal for every great medical biller – first time, every time.**

Now this is not always easy because how a CMS 1500 claim form is completed will differ. Every carrier is different and what they expect the claim to look like can vary. Some carriers want minimal information on the claim form while others require that almost every field on the form have some data.

The company I work for is nationwide, so I deal with every type of health insurance plan. In order to keep track of the various requirements per carrier, I keep a BIG binder of "cheat sheets." I refer to these cheat sheets on a daily basis to provide me with special billing information. *Special,* to me, is any special instructions, required attachments, EDI Submitter numbers, required modifiers, etc. This way I am confident that I have what I need to submit a clean claim. If the billing process is simple, a cheat sheet is not necessary. However, some carriers have more than one cheat sheet, for example:

- Carriers that operate in different states, like Blue Cross Blue Shield.
- Carriers that handle different plan types, United HealthCare handles commercial, Medicare and Medicaid plans so I tend to make one for each plan type.

Remember, a claim tells a story about the patient and nobody likes to have pages of the story missing. We all want to know the when, where, why, what and how in every story and claim billing is really no different.

A Clean Claim Includes:

- Who is the patient?
- Where does the patient live?
- Who is the provider that performed the service?
- Where is the provider located?
- What health plan information does the patient have?
- What services are being performed?
- When was the visit?
- Why is the patient being seen?
- How old are they?
- How much did the visit cost?
- What modifier do I need to bill?
- What documentation should accompany the claim?
- What are the correct codes?

All of these questions, if answered correctly on your billed claim, should result in this claim moving through the insurance process without being held, rejected or denied.

How to Ensure that Your Claim is Clean.

- Do your homework. Find out what the health carrier requires before your first claim is submitted. You can call the health carrier or go online at the carrier's website.

- The first instinct, when a claim is not paid, is to simply rebill it. Don't! Call the carrier first and find out exactly why the claim was not paid.
- Make yourself a billing manual that includes all of the special tips and tricks you have learned, by trial and error. This will include billing address changes, special modifiers, special instructions, etc. This way you don't have to reinvent the wheel when you are faced with a claim issue.

So where did the term clean claim come from? I am not sure who coined the phrase but I am guessing it was a health insurance carrier. Health carriers are quick to proclaim that the primary reason that claims are denied or paid incorrectly is due to billing errors.

From Experience

When account receivables starts to rise, everyone takes notice and the common assumption is that either:

1. Claims are not being billed, or
2. Claims are not being billed correctly.

Let me add number 3, health insurance carriers make errors and lots of them. Some of those errors include:

- Claims paid out of network in error.
- Lost claims.
- Supporting data that was submitted with the claim, but somehow is missing
- Overlooked authorization numbers, referring provider information, etc.
- Incorrect claim payments and denials.

Yes, a clean claim is critical, but it is only half of the process. ***Errors occur on both sides.*** Taking the extra steps to make sure your claim meets the clean claim standard is critical. But errors do occur which is why you also have to keep your eye on A/R and if a claim is not paid, call the health carrier for status.

For difficult claims where I've had to bill it more than once before it was paid, I also keep a copy of the claim with the patient info removed so I have an example of how to recreate it the next time.

Health carriers have started to return claims that have billing errors. Review all returned claims for more than just address corrections.

Take the time to read the many health carrier bulletins you receive, they provide "advanced warning" about billing changes, new procedures, required modifiers, etc., so you can incorporate this information into your billed claims early to avoid rejects.

ASSIGNMENT OF BENEFITS

One of the main questions that needs to be answered when billing a claim is:

Who should get paid?

The CMS 1500 claim form is where you would tell the insurance carrier where the payment should go. The health insurance carrier will use the information that the medical biller enters on the claim form as a means to instruct them how they should issue the payment for the claim, either to the patient or to the medical provider directly.

Box 13 on the CMS 1500 claim form is where you make that designation.

Box 13 of the CMS form states "Insured or Authorized Person's Signature: I authorize payment of medical benefits to the undersigned physician or supplier for services described below."

Assigned billing means that all payments related to that claim will be **paid to the physician or supplier**. This is accomplished by having the signature of the authorized person in box 13 of the CMS 1500 form.

Unassigned billing means all payments related to that claim will be **paid to the patient**. This is accomplished by leaving box 13 of the CMS 1500 form blank.

Because the patient would have left the office when the CMS form is created, a "live" patient signature is usually not possible. To solve the problem of not having the patient available when a claim needs to be billed, the provider's office will have the authorized person sign an Assignment of Benefit form (AOB) when they are in the office.

This signed Assignment of Benefit form will remain in the patient's file unless revoked. To revoke, simply means to cancel the form out. The patient will contact the provider's office to let them know that they want to change the Assignment of Benefit form that they have on file. The old form will be replaced with the new and future claims will be handled in accordance with the new form.

Because a signed AOB form is on file, the notation "SIGNATURE ON FILE" is placed in Box 13 of the CMS 1500 form, instead of a signature. This means that in lieu of a signature, written permission is on file to have all payments made to the provider of service.

Failure to have a signed AOB form on file means that Box 13 must be left blank and all payments will be made to the patient.

In order for claims payments to be issued correctly, two things have to happen:

- The Medical Biller is responsible for checking to make sure that all claims have the proper assignment; the CMS 1500 form must have the correct information in Box 13.
- The health carrier must pay the claims based on the information that is in Box 13.

Box 13 may not be the only factor that affects the assignment of benefits, the carrier may have some rules that apply.

For Example:

- In network providers are usually paid directly, in spite of the assignment.
- Out of network provider benefits are usually paid to the patient in spite of the assignment.
- Facility services, like hospitals, are usually paid to the facility.

Any doubt, call the health carrier to confirm how the claim will be paid.

CLEARINGHOUSE

The patient is seen by the provider and a claim that details the visit is created and uploaded to a batch file that is submitted, either automatically or manually, to an outside entity called a clearinghouse. A batch file is a file that contains all of the claims that you created for submission to the insurance carrier and condenses them into a single file. Most claims submitted electronically will go through a clearinghouse because most billing systems lack the ability to translate every claim to the correct format that each insurance carrier may need.

So what is a Clearinghouse?

In medical billing, the middleman between the provider and the insurance carrier is called a clearinghouse. A clearinghouse's role is to:

- ***Scrub the claim*** by checking for errors and verifying that the claim is compatible with the payer software.
- Implement policies and procedures that protect electronic Protected Health Information (PHI) from unauthorized access and is responsible for reporting any breach of data to the affected parties in order to comply with HIPAA requirements.
- Provide a service to both providers and insurance carriers by ensuring faster more accurate

submission of claims, EOB's and payments. Both will pay the clearinghouse for the service they provide. Both will be enrolled to send and receive claims.

- Ensure claims that go through the clearinghouse will have an electronic date stamp that shows the date the claim was transmitted and the date the claim was accepted by the health carrier. This is the assurance that the claim is on file at the health plan and that it has passed the clearinghouse edits.

Once the claim is transmitted to the Clearinghouse, the claim will be checked for errors. If errors are found, the claim will be returned back to the medical biller for correction and then resubmission.

Some of the edits that a Clearinghouse could check for are:

- The ID number is correct.
- The procedural and diagnosis codes are correct.
- The procedure being performed fits the diagnosis.
- The relationship to the subscriber is correct.
- The patient's name and date of birth is correct.
- The COB calculations are correct.
- You are properly enrolled to submit claims electronically to that carrier.
- You are submitting to the correct carrier.
- The carrier accepts electronic secondary claims.

Claims with errors need to be fixed immediately

- If the claim is not corrected and resubmitted, it will remain in a holding pattern, unprocessed and aging until some human takes the time to review it.
- The health carrier will have no record of these claims because they would have been returned prior to reaching the health carrier.

- Fixing an error could be as simple as correcting the spelling on the patient's name, calling the patient for updated insurance information, or it could be a claim that cannot be submitted electronically, requiring billing by paper.

The way to fix the error will vary but ALL errors should be fixed daily.

Please be aware that an error free claim does not guarantee that the claim will be paid nor does it mean that this same claim will be deemed error free by the health carrier. Most health carriers will subject a claim to a wide range of additional edits.

Clearinghouses not only submit claims but most have a host of other services such as eligibility verification, paper claim submission, patient invoicing and revenue management.

ELECTRONIC VS. PAPER CLAIMS

When I started in this industry, years ago, we used a typewriter to complete claim forms and ***every claim*** was submitted on paper. Today, paper submission of claims is becoming a thing of the past with providers submitting most claims electronically.

We still have some situations where EDI falls short, especially in situations when we do not have the option to upload data to accompany the claim. For example, claims for secondary or tertiary billing where an EOB is required to determine the plan's liability, claims where additional information is required to support medical necessity like letters, test results and operative reports, and claims where an invoice is needed for claim pricing. However, there is really no comparison when you begin to look at the pros and cons of each.

Paper Claims

- Paper claims are slow and cumbersome and can be hard to complete. The data has to fit squarely in the field. The ink can't be too light to prevent front end scanning. Some fonts are hard to read and some claims cannot be folded, requiring the use of large, more costly, envelopes and postage.
- Until the claim is scanned by the health carrier into their system, which could take days to complete, you have NO idea if the claim even reached its destination. Lost claims are a normal part of the

paper claim submission process. There is nothing as frustrating as waiting weeks for a claim to be processed only to be told they do not have record of ever receiving the claim. The claim must then be rebilled and the waiting game must be started all over again.

- The claim is created and mailed to the health carrier and for some reason it is misdirected or lost and your Protected Health Information (PHI) ends up in the hands of someone who really does not need to know where you live, your phone number or what you are being treated for.

EDI

Clearly, Electronic Data Interchange (EDI) has a number of benefits over billing paper.

- EDI claims are delivered much faster than paper; in a matter of hours instead of the days that it takes for the claim to reach the insurance carrier by mail.
- NO lost or misdirected claims. EDI provides an automated date stamp that shows when the claim was received. This is critical when trying to dispute timely filing denials.
- Claims submitted electronically are usually paid earlier than paper claims.
- Claims submitted electronically are sent to a clearinghouse where they are subject to some edit and error detection processes that are designed to make you fix any problems with the claim before it goes to be processed.
- Claims submitted electronically have lower overall costs. EDI eliminates the need for postage; bulk orders of CMS 1500 claims forms, envelopes, printer paper and ink cartridges.
- Claims submitted electronically can also have claim payments and an EOB/Remittance Advice submitted electronically as well. This means faster secondary billing, posting of payments, patient invoices and account reconciliation.
- EDI is a much safer, HIPAA compliant, way to submit claims.

WHAT YOU NEED FROM THE PATIENT

It really does take a village- the patient, the provider and the health carrier, to get a claim from initial encounter to electronic payment (or paper check).

You will you need:

- A copy of the patient's insurance identification card front and back.
- Completed health history forms.
- HIPAA forms that clearly state the office privacy policy including how the Protected Health Information (PHI) will be handled.
- A completed Assignment of Benefits form with a signature of the patient or guardian authorizing the insurance carrier to pay the doctor, not the patient, for all billed services.
- A completed Release of Information form with a signature of the patient or guardian giving the provider the permission to release information about the patient's medical condition and treatment to anyone with the need to know. The types of people that would ***need to know*** would be the insurance carrier, any specialists etc.
- A completed Advanced Beneficiary Notice (ABN) form with a signature from a Medicare beneficiary when you have reason to believe that Medicare may not pay for the service that you are rendering to

the patient. This form advises the patient of any potentially service that is not covered and by signature they can indicate whether they want to proceed with the service and whether to bill Medicare. No ABN is needed for services that you know are not covered by Medicare.

- Patients who are willing to jump in, arms swinging, to help resolve any issue that may affect the provider's and, ultimately, the patient's pocket.

Patients Are Our Best Resource

I believe that patients should have the kind of relationship with their health care providers that promote comfort, communication and confidence. All expectations should be clear, from both sides, with no surprises. Patients should be kept in the loop regarding any issue that affects their healthcare or their health insurance.

Patients can be the best resource when you have hit a brick wall on an unresolved claim issue. One call from the patient may help you to:

- Move a claim from pending to payment.
- Resolve a payment problem or dispute.
- Solve a plan, benefit or coverage issue.

A bit of pressure from the patient may work the magic that is needed to finally get that problem claim resolved. Health insurance carriers do not like to have unhappy, "I am going to complain about your service to my HR," type of plan members because that may affect business.

Real world example

A very young patient, with medical issues, was in urgent need of some extensive therapy. The parents are divorced and the child resides with the mom. The divorce decree mandated that the father's coverage be primary and the mom's coverage be secondary.

We had contacted both health carriers, in advance, and was granted out of network approval from the dad's plan and in net approval from the mom's plan. The services were performed and the dad's plan was billed.

Weeks later, I call to check status on this unpaid claim and learn that a payment of $4200.00 was made directly to the dad. Because we are an out of network provider, the health carrier refused to provide a copy of the EOB or to provide any other details about this claim.

I contacted the mom for assistance, informing her that we needed two things: the $4200.00 payment and the EOB so that I could bill the secondary plan for the balance. She contacted her ex-husband and ***yes*** he had received the check and ***no*** he did not have the money as he used it to put a down payment on a new truck. He also refused to provide a copy of the EOB to mom.

Mom asked that I give her three months to get this resolved. I agreed and her account was flagged for follow up in 90 days.

About 2 months later, the mom called me back. She had sued her ex-husband and because of the child's medical needs, was granted an emergency hearing. Not only was dad ordered to pay the $4200.00 payment immediately and provide us with a copy of the EOB, he ended up paying all of her court costs and was threatened with jail time if this happened again.

This issue would never have been resolved had the mom not jumped in to help. Resolution was critical so that further access to care was not affected.

WHAT EVERY CLAIM NEEDS

The initial patient encounter is where you would make sure that you have ***everything that is needed*** to move from visit to billing to payment. Having everything you need, before the patient leaves the office, helps to create that clean claim that should be processed quickly and accurately by the health insurance carrier.

How to ensure you have everything you need to get this claim paid

Step One - Although the patient may have provided enough information to secure a spot on the calendar, once they are in the office we need the hardcopy information that is needed to create a file for the patient and start the process.

The Information:

- Plan type: Medicare, Medicaid, Tricare, Group plan, other
- The patient demographics: name, age, date of birth, address, phone number.
- The health carrier information, such as relationship to patient, plan holder name and date of birth, employer name and address, group numbers and correct ID numbers.
- If other coverage exists and, if so, the complete plan name, address, and ID numbers of any secondary or tertiary carrier.

- If the condition is related to an injury, or is work related.
- Referring provider name and NPI information.
- Correct ICD indicator (ICD-9 or ICD-10)
- The correct ICD-10, CPT, and/or HCPCS coding and the correct charges.
- Correct provider of service information. Including correct provider numbers, NPI and service location.
- Patient's "signature on file" authorizing release of information as well as authorizing the insurance carrier to pay either the patient or the provider directly.
- Correct place of service code.
- Correct Prior Authorization number.
- Correct dates of service.
- Correct charge for each service
- Correct number of items or units
- Correct modifier if needed.
- All supporting information including: operative reports, letters of medical necessity, primary carrier's EOB's, invoices, etc. (The time it takes for the carrier to request additional information and for you to respond may take months.)

Step Two - Now that we have the plan information, step two is all about turning this piece of paper into a positive confirmation of coverage. This will then allow you to take this from a billed charge to a fully paid claim.

The Process

- Call the health carrier to verify benefits and eligibility on all new patients, every time. For returning patients, call again if it has been more than a month.

- Collect all amounts deemed to be a patient's portion upfront.
- Secure needed referral or preapprovals on all required services, treatments and supplies. Make sure you have this as a hardcopy not just verbally.
- Always code to the highest level of specificity. Especially with the new ICD-10 codes that were expanded to include a wider ranges of codes to choose from. Make sure that the person that is responsible for pre-coding all claims is not just cross walking from the old ICD-9 code to the exact same ICD-10 code. Coders should be taking the time to review the new ICD-10 manual to select the exact code/s that best fits the claim.
- Set yourself up to bill claims electronically whenever possible. Most health carriers have an enrollment process that, once completed, will allow you to bill electronically and also receive electronic (EFT) payments and online EOB's and Remittance Advices.
- A signed ABN form for all Medicare beneficiaries for service, supplies or treatment that may not be paid by Medicare. Do not accept the patient's assurance that they understand a service may not be covered. Failure to have a signed ABN will work in the patient's favor and you may be required to refund back any monies collected.

Finally, never assume that the carrier has all of the information on file. The responsibility is on the biller to get it right not on the claim payer to piece your billed claim together.

COORDINATION OF BENEFITS

Coordination of Benefits (COB) is the process of determining how claims will be processed when a patient has two or more health insurance carriers. The primary carrier will pay first and the secondary carrier may pick up the balance. This additional coverage may be available because:

- A spouse also has health coverage through their employer.
- A person has two jobs and two coverages.
- Two working parents each insure a child under an employer plan.
- Government plans like Medicare or Medicaid.
- Medigap plans.
- Military plans.

Determining the order is important because it enables you to understand which carrier should be billed first, how claims will be reimbursed and if the patient will have any out of pocket costs.

Most health plans are written so that plan members share in the cost of healthcare. For example, an 80/20 plan means that a carrier will pay 80% of the covered charges leaving the patient to pay the remaining 20%. When a patient has more than one plan, all health plans will be billed and all payments will be applied to that date of service.

Example 1 of COB

Ben J. has an 80/20 plan through his place of employment and his wife, Janis J, also covers him under an 80/20 plan through her company. Neither plan has a deductible.

Ben goes to the doctor and incurs $500.00 in healthcare costs.

BEN'S PLAN:

Allowed Amount: $500.00

Benefit: $500.00 x (80%) = $400.00

Ben's plan pays $400.00 leaving him a balance of $100.00

The same claim is billed to Janis' plan with the EOB showing the $400.00 payment.

JANIS' PLAN:

Allowed Amount: $500.00

Benefit: $500.00 x (80%) = $400.00

Although Janis's plan could pay out $400.00, they know that the bill was only $500.00 and that $400.00 has already been paid by the primary carrier. They issue a payment for $100.00. Between the two carriers the claim has been paid in full with ZERO out of pocket from the patient.

Keep in mind that each carrier will only pay up to its allowed amounts. Let's look at an example of this.

Example 2 of COB

Sally M. has a Blue Cross 80/20 PPO plan as primary and a Medicaid plan that pays 100% of allowed as secondary. Sally goes to an in network doctor and incurs $1000.00 in medical costs.

The claim is billed to the primary plan Blue Cross first:

SALLY'S BLUE CROSS PLAN:

Billed: $1000.00

Blue Cross Allowed: $800.00

Blue Cross Paid: $640.00 ($800 x 80%)

Balance is $160.00 ($800.00 x 20%)
($200.00 is adjusted as over allowed amount.)

The secondary Medicaid plan is billed:

SALLY'S MEDICAID PLAN:

Billed: $1000.00
Medicaid Allowed: $500.00
Since the primary carrier paid more than Medicaid allowed, they will pay zero.

The balance of $160.00 is deemed to be over Medicaid allowed and will be adjusted off.

In a Nutshell

- In spite of how the clam is calculated, no more than 100% of the billed charge will be paid.
- The health carrier deemed to be the primary carrier is billed first.
- Both carriers CANNOT be billed at the same time.
- The primary carrier will determine their liability and the EOB, from this determination, will be used to bill the secondary carrier. Unless you have a way to attach the EOB electronically, your secondary claim will be billed as a paper claim.
- Even if we know in advance that the primary carrier will deny coverage for a service or supply, we must still bill them because we will need that denial in order to bill the secondary.
- When you call the health carrier, you may not learn about a second or third coverage but if you handle all benefits and eligibility verification through an online system you may have access to information on any and all health carriers that a patient has.
- Patients with more than one health carrier do not get to decide not to use one. They are required to disclose all information about all health plans so that claims can be handled correctly.

Real World Example

A few years ago, we had a patient that filled out the insurance forms indicating that she had Medicaid coverage only. She provides us with the front and back of her Medicaid ID card, we call to verify benefits and eligibility and since preapproval was not required the service is provided and the claim was billed.

Shortly after, Medicaid denies her claim because she has other primary coverage. We contact the patient who says she, "does not want to use that coverage." She feels that it is her right not to use a carrier. After numerous attempts, she still refused to fully disclose her primary plan and Medicaid refused to honor our claim that ended up aging out. Thankfully, we now have systems in place for situations such as these.

TIMELY FILING

You create a claim and mail it to the health carrier for processing and 90 days later, no payment, no denial, nothing. So you call the insurance carrier to check status and you learn that, for whatever reason, your claim was never received; they have no record of the claim.

So, you create another claim and mail it to the health carrier. Because the first claim went missing, you call the health carrier 14 days later and the health carrier confirms that, yes, they have the claim on file. You add this to the "win" category since payment is surely on the way. A few weeks later you receive a letter stating that the claim has been denied for timely filing.

You call the carrier and learn that this plan has a 60 day timely filing period. You have 60 days from the date the service was rendered to get that claim over to the health carrier. Your claim was initially billed well within that time frame but you have no proof that the claim was ever received by the carrier. No payment will be forthcoming on this claim.

What is time filing?

Timely filing refers to the amount of time you have to get that claim over to the health carrier. Timely filing periods vary greatly. I have seen some as short as 30 days and some as long as 365 days. 365 days is average but more and more carriers are moving toward 180 days and shorter timely filing periods. ***This refers to mailed claims only since electronic claims will have an automatic time tracking.*** Claims received by the health carrier after the timely filing period will be denied as "too old" to process.

Example of timely filing:

Timely filing period: 60 days

Claim date of service: 1/1/16

Claim received: 3/10/16

Claim will be denied

If a claim is denied for time filing you really do not have much recourse. So, the plan is to be proactive and not reactive, for example:

- Find out the timely filing period from the health carrier's website or from Customer Service when you call to verify benefits and eligibility.
- Bill electronically, this way you have an automatic date stamp that shows when your claim was received by the health carrier. You can use this to dispute all timely filing denials.
- Keep cheat sheets of all timely filing periods or, at the very least, the ones that have short filing periods.
- Calendar to make sure that you call the health carrier to confirm that the claim has been received for all health plans that have a short timely filing period.
- Keep your eye on all secondary or tertiary claims, as the clock will start ticking from the date of the primary/secondary EOB, not the date you decide to bill the claim.
- Timely filing periods also affect the time you have to dispute an incorrect claim payment.

Unless the patient is clearly at fault for failing to provide some necessary information that was needed to bill the claim, maybe the patient failed to provide a copy of the primary carrier's EOB or an updated insurance ID card; you will have a hard time making the patient responsible for the balance that remains on account because the provider's office failed to get the claim over to the carrier timely.

Most timely filing errors are usually written off as bad debt, meaning the patient is not billed and the provider's revenue will take a hit for any claims that cannot be reimbursed.

CHAPTER FIVE TEST

Directions: Using what you have learned in Chapter Five, answer the following questions.

1. What does it mean to submit a clean claim?

2. What purpose does an AOB form serve?

3. What information goes into box 13 on the CMS form?

4. What does the phrase ***scrub a claim*** refer to?

5. What is the point of Coordination of Benefits?

6. There is not a signed AOB on file but the provider is in network, who will receive the payment?

7. What does the term batch file mean?

8. What does HIPAA have to do with a clearinghouse?

9. Why is a release of information form needed?

10. Can a patient be balance billed if the biller failed to submit a claim timely?

6 CLAIM JOURNEY

Chapter Overview – Where does a claim go after it is submitted? In this chapter, we provide a step-by-step look at the insurance process; starting from the patient's initial call to schedule an appointment up until when final payment is posted.

This Chapter Includes:

FOLLOW THAT CLAIM

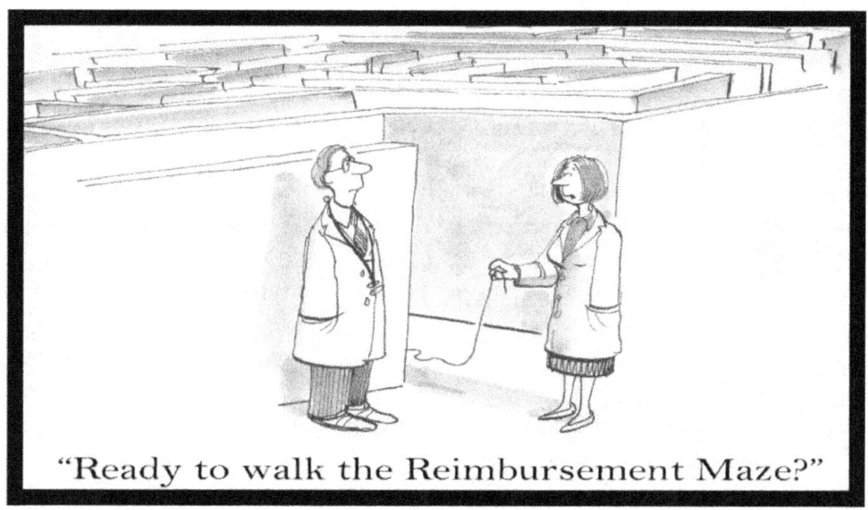
"Ready to walk the Reimbursement Maze?"

A look at the claim's process from first encounter to final resolution.

Day 1 - A new patient calls the doctor's office requesting an appointment to see the doctor. While on the phone, they are asked to provide some personal information including the full name and date of birth of the patient and the reason for the visit. If insured, they also must provide the patient's identification and group numbers and the name and contact numbers of their health insurance carrier. The appointment is scheduled.

Day 5 - Prior to the scheduled visit, the patient's health carrier will be contacted by phone or online, to confirm eligibility and to determine benefits, plan type, coverage details and if the plan has any preapproval or referral requirements.

The doctor's office will use this information to try to determine how a health carrier may pay for the visit. The patient will be required to pay any charges that may not be reimbursed by the health carrier. They will also facilitate any upfront preapprovals or referrals that may be required.

Day 6 – Once the patient is in the office, they will be asked to complete the necessary health history forms, sign the Assignment of Benefits (AOB), Release of Information, HIPAA and Privacy forms and provide copies of his/her driver's license and insurance cards and pay any applicable upfront costs.

Once they see the doctor, all aspects of the visit will be documented, maybe in real time using some type of EHR/EMR system. A detailed accounting of the reason for the visit will be listed, including but not limited to: chief complaints, patient and family history, vaccines, all medications, any needed referrals, the current diagnosis, treatment and testing as well as any recommendations for management of the current condition.

Detailed documentation is mandatory as it ensures proper coding of the claim, serves to validate that all tests and treatments are fully supported in the patient's file and will satisfy any applicable quality reporting requirements.

The patient will leave the office with an encounter form that details the diagnoses and services that were provided.

Day 7 - Using the documentation from the visit, the correct ICD-10, CPT-4, HCPCS codes and provider fees will be assigned.

The doctor will be asked to review the patient's history to assign the correct codes for any unique, unusual or complex visits or where a valid code does not exist.

Day 8 - Using some type of billing software, a CMS 1500 form, detailing this encounter, will be created. The CMS 1500 form will include all of the codes, charges documentation and patient information, as supported in the patient's file, that is needed to bill a clean claim to the carrier.

Electronic claims will go into a batch file to be uploaded to the clearinghouse.

Paper claims are printed with supporting documents attached (if needed) and mailed to the health carrier.

Day 9 - Electronic claims have reached the Clearinghouse where they are checked for basic errors. Error free claims will be transmitted on to the health carrier to start claim processing. Claims with errors will be kicked back to the biller for correction and resubmission.

Day 10 - 45 – The claim adjudication process will vary greatly. On average, a claim is processed 20 - 45 days from the date it is received - but again this will vary greatly.

A lot of factors affect how long it *really* takes for a claim to be processed by the health insurance carrier including: the method of claim delivery (paper vs electronic), the health carrier's current claim backlog, EFT vs paper checks and even by the type of service or procedure code as some may require more time for review and pricing.

But before this process can begin, the claim must have first reached the health carrier. Electronic claims will be transmitted directly from the clearinghouse to the health carrier. Paper claims require each envelope to be delivered, opened, and with all supporting documents attached, scanned into the system for easy retrieval.

The claim will be assigned to a Claim Processor who will run it through the claim processing system to:

- Confirm that the patient is eligible.
- Determine how the patient's benefits and plan provisions will apply to that claim.
- Determine that the claim has been submitted correctly.
- Determine that the claim has been billed to the correct payer.
- Determine the status of the provider
- Subject the claim to numerous edits. Edits can be made for correct coding, any fraud indicators or suspect billing, appropriateness of charges, validity of codes, correct place of service, any unbundling, units or day limits, investigation or experimental services, age limits, plan provisions or any other edits that the health carrier deems necessary.
- Determine how the claim should be priced. Pricing is based on whatever methodology applies i.e. contracted rate, Medicare fee schedule, Medicaid fee schedule, UCR or any other method as determined by the health carrier.
- Determine that the claim has all of the information needed to complete processing.
- Determine method of reimbursement, EFT or paper.
- Create an EOB.
- Issue a letter, either to the patient, the provider or both, requesting additional information needed to complete processing.

At ANY point the claim could be rejected and returned for correction, pended for additional information or flat out denied.

In reality, most Claim Processors simply do not have the high level of expertise needed to effectively process all types of health claims. This is why the true MVP is the Claim Processing System. The average claim will go through a maze of different hurdles before it is deemed payable. So, a good claim processing system must:

- Be able to accept a claim no matter what format it is submitted.

- Have the logic that is needed to shift through thousands of names, some very similar, to pull up the exact patient that applies to that claim.
- Have the logic needed to shift through thousands of plans, some very similar, to pull up the exact plan that applies to that claim.
- Contain thousands of tables and decision charts so it provides the logic needed to determine that the billed code: fits the diagnosis for the correct part of the body, is performed in the correct setting and by the correct provider type and is appropriate based on the accepted standards of care.
- Have the logic needed to pull up the appropriate provider, finalize payment, either EFT or paper, and generate an EOB that displays the correct coding that exactly matches the way the claim was handled.
- Have the ability to store and report on all data so that one can easily segregate and monitor any and all industry changes or trends, suspect providers or procedures, high level claims, new technologies, etc.

Once the claim clears processing:

- A Remittance Advice/EOB and payment (if applicable) will be issued either electronically (EFT) or by paper check, to the provider of service; if the claim was assigned. A paper check will be mailed to the patient for all unassigned claims.
- A letter will be generated asking the provider or the patient to provide any and all information that is needed to complete processing, including: medical records, history and physical, test results, invoices, authorizations, referrals, other insurance information, etc. The claim may be closed, pended or denied until the required information is provided.
- A letter will be generated that explains the reason the claim was denied and the appeal options.

The Goal is Zero Due on Account

Once the check has been received, then it will be up to the doctor's office to post all payments to the account and review ALL EOB/RA's to determine if the claim processed as expected. Even EOB/RA's with zero payments will be reviewed since they provide a piece of the payment puzzle.

If ZERO on account is not met:

- The claim will corrected and rebilled.
- The claim be disputed or appealed.
- Additional information will be provided to support coverage.
- The health carrier will be contacted to provide clarification on how the claim was processed.
- A statement will be sent to the patient for the balance.
- The balance will be written off.
- The secondary (tertiary) carrier will be billed.

Finally, timely follow-up on all open balances is needed until the claim is resolved.

Summary

This section provides a realistic overview of how a claim is really handled - starting from the patient's first call for appointment to how the heath carrier may actually adjudicate the claim to, finally, zero due on account.

Keep in mind the days and the process will vary. Electronic claims tend to move faster through the system while paper claims add days to the process and you have no assurance that the claim is even on file unless you contact the carrier.

This overview in no way suggests that the process is one size fits all, that it is simple or easy, predictable or even that billing always results in quick payment. The goal of zero balance on account may be bumpy and time consuming and may draw on all aspects of your insurance expertise and experience.

CHAPTER SIX TEST

Directions: Using what you have learned in Chapter Six, answer the following questions.

1. Summarize, in your own words, the typical process of a claim. Use detail to support your answer.

2. What is the single most important take way from Chapter 6? Explain in detail.

7 REIMBURSEMENT

Chapter Overview - The ultimate goal of a Medical Biller is to use their expertise to make sure that every claim is adequately reimbursed. In this chapter, we will look at the various aspects related to payment.

This Chapter Includes:

Contracted Rates

Usual, Customary & Reasonable

Allowed Amounts

Medicare Fee Schedule

Medicaid Fee Schedule

EFT vs. Paper Checks

Write Offs/Adjustments

Collecting Upfront

EOB/Remittance Advice

Appeals/Disputes

Revenue Management

CONTRACTED RATES

Dr. Smith decides to become part of a commercial health carrier's network of participating providers of all specialties. He contacts the health carrier, goes through the enrollment and credentialing process, agrees to the terms of participation and, once completed, his name is added to the provider directory.

Using the provider directory, a patient selects Dr. Smith and calls his office for an appointment. Because commercial health insurance carriers, unlike Medicare and Medicaid, do not publish fee schedules that list the allowed amounts for all services by CPT-4 code, Dr. Smith's office does not have an exact way to determine what the patient is required to pay upfront nor will they know for certain what he may be reimbursed.

The services are provided to the patient and the claim is billed using the provider's normal charge for all services. The health carrier will then re-price each billed charge to the contracted rate that is on file for the provider.

What is a Contracted Rate?

One of the key provisions that a provider must agree to, once they become participating providers, is the acceptance of the health insurance carrier's contracted rate. Carriers use contracted rates to reimburse providers for services rendered to members covered under a managed care plan. This use of contracted rates allows health carriers to manage costs because a participating provider is usually paid less than his normally billed charges.

Health insurance carriers use contracted rates to determine what will be allowed and ultimately paid on a billed claim. Contracted rates could use a flat amount for each service, a percentage discount, or some other methodology. Reimbursement is usually less than the amount that a provider normally would charge for that same service.

A contracted rate is agreed upon, by contract, between the provider and the insurance carrier in advance.

Participating providers accept the contracted rate and agree not to balance bill the patient for any charges that exceed these rates. Patients would be responsible for any applicable copay, deductible and coinsurance amounts only.

Example

DR. SMITH BILLS THE FOLLOWING:

$100.00 (Office Visit)

+ $100.00 (Chest X-Ray)

$200.00 Total Billed

The insurance company applies the contracted rate and determines that they will allow the following:

CARRIER ALLOWS THE FOLLOWING:

$50.00 (Office Visit)

+ $50.00 (Chest X-Ray)

$100.00 Total Allowed

$100.00 is not covered as it is over the contracted rate and will be adjusted off by the provider.

So your next question may be why would any doctor accept such a reduction in billed charges? The answer is simple:

Today, most patients have some type of managed care plan and if a doctor wants to keeps their practice profitable they need to treat a steady stream of patients. Healthcare is expensive and managed care plans are designed to require low or no money out of pocket for patients that choose to see a participating provider. This means that a provider may have better access to more patients with all kinds of different plan types if they participate.

USUAL, CUSTOMARY & REASONABLE

Health insurance carriers may use Usual, Customary and Reasonable rates (UCR) as a way to determine how much to reimburse a provider for services rendered to members that are covered under traditional (fee for service) and out of network plans.

Do not assume that just because a provider is considered non-participating that the health carrier will accept any amount that a provider chooses to bill for a service. Every claim processed by a health insurance carrier will go through some type of re-pricing, whether they use contracted rates for participating providers or UCR for non-participating providers.

The UCR rate is the maximum allowable that a carrier will reimburse for a particular service, regardless of what the provider may bill for that same service. The health carrier considers the UCR rate to be the "normal or average charge" for a service. Each CPT code that is billed will have a UCR amount tied to it.

The Problem with UCR is that:

- The methodology for determining the UCR rate is hard to figure out. In order to predict the UCR amount, you would have to poll all like providers in the same area, using the same billing codes, who are willing to release their fees for comparison.

- UCR rates are not usually disclosed up front nor are their rates published anywhere. Providers and patients have no way to plan for the potential out of pocket costs.
- UCR rates may differ from insurance carrier to insurance carrier, so no "standard" reimbursement exists.

If UCR is applied on a non-managed care plan, the portion deemed over UCR can be billed and collected directly from the patient or from a secondary carrier. The patient would also be responsible for any deductible and coinsurance amounts.

This "normal/average charge" is a combination of:

- The usual fee charged for that service.
- What providers in the same geographic area are customarily charging for that same service.
- Taking into account any reasonable and extenuating circumstances.

The result is the amount that will be considered the allowed amount for that charge.

For Example

Dr. Smith, Dr. James and Dr. Jones all practice in Los Angeles, California, all are pediatricians and all have offices within a few miles of each other.

Dr. Smith bills $300.00 for an initial newborn exam.

Dr. James bills $250.00 for an initial newborn exam.

Dr. Jones bills $250.00 for an initial newborn exam.

The health plan takes into consideration what all like providers are billing for this same service and they will use this data to come with a "usual" charge. Using the example above, both Dr. James and Dr. Jones bill the same amount for a newborn exam among providers located in that area of Los Angeles, California, so the health carrier could determine that the "usual" rate for an initial newborn exam will be $250.00.

Dr. Smith's claim is over the UCR rate so it will be reduced to $250.00. The claims from Dr. James and Dr. Jones will be accepted as billed with no reduction. ***Note: this represents a general overview of how UCR may be determined. Every carrier is different so use this as a guide to understanding the process.***

Since most carriers lack the time and expertise to figure out the UCR computation for thousands of CPT-4 codes, as well as to continuously update them as needed, they may purchase a software program from an outside vendor that provides this information. This program is loaded into their system and will read each CPT-4 code and apply the correct allowable amounts. This information is normally updated annually.

Example

The following example illustrates how UCR may be applied.

DR. SMITH BILLS THE FOLLOWING:

$100.00 (Office Visit)

+ $50.00 (Chest X-Ray)

$150.00 Total Billed

The insurance company applies the UCR allowance and determines that they will only allow the following:

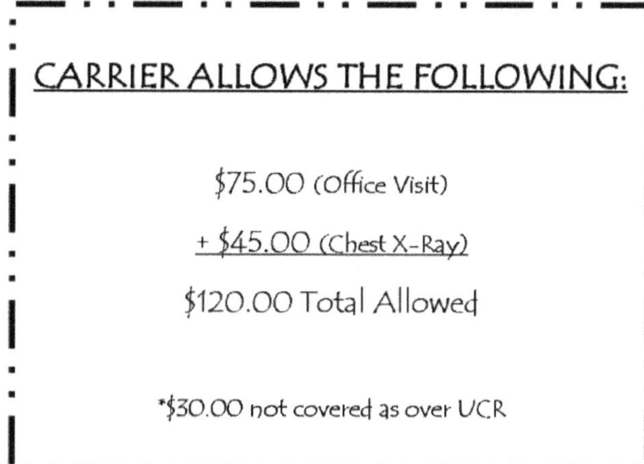

Using this example, the provider will not be reimbursed as billed and the patient can expect to incur more out-of-pocket expenses.

ALLOWED AMOUNTS

All throughout this guide, you have seen the term "allowed amount" mentioned over and over again. Allowed amount is that totally misunderstood, totally hard to predict, totally critical piece of the pie that brings everything into focus.

So what does allowed amount really mean?

If you have ever filed an insurance claim, be it homeowners, auto or health, you know that the amount you think should be paid and the amount the insurance carrier thinks the claim is valued at are usually two totally different amounts.

Medical providers spend a lot of time setting the rates and fees for each of the services that they perform and the CMS 1500 claim is billed to the carrier with these carefully selected billed amounts.

Once the health carrier receives that claim, that billed amount is "re-priced" to an amount that the carrier deems payable for that claim.

That amount is deemed to be the allowed amount.

Every health carrier has a different methodology for determining which portion of that billed amount is considered eligible for coverage. The steps to determining allowed amounts could be tough to figure out. Any of the numerous methods could apply as determined by the health carrier and, in the case of managed care plans, as agreed to by the provider. Each method could differ by carrier and even by plan type. Some of these methods include:

- Capitation
- Usual, Customary & Reasonable
- Fee Schedule
- Billed Amount
- Any other methods

The bottom line is that you should always have some idea how the claim will be processed by the health plan. Allowed amount is critical to revenue management as it helps you to understand what portion of the billed amount will be paid.

Keep a cheat sheet, by carrier, of the allowed amounts for your most common procedures this way you have some idea what to collect up front and what you will have to adjust off on the back end.

Knowing how much of the billed claim you expect to be considered for reimbursement will allow you to:

- Determine what to collect upfront.
- Determine if the claim was paid correctly.
- Determine if you need to dispute or appeal the payment.
- Determine if you need to balance bill the patient.

- Determine the amount to adjust off.
- Determine if you need to bill a secondary carrier.

And on a higher level, it helps the provider of service to understand if the decision to participate with a particular network is yielding the results needed to maintain that relationship or, at the very least, try to renegotiate the contract for better reimbursement.

The allowed amount is usually less than what the provider bills for that same service. So it is important to keep an eye on payments so you can anticipate and keep track of reimbursement.

For Example

A doctor bills $100.00 for an exam and $25.00 for a blood test. The health carrier reduces the billed amount to $50 for the exam and $10.00 for the blood test.

The allowed amount is $50.00 for the exam and $10.00 for the blood test.

The claim is now processed as if the claim was billed for $60.00 instead of the $125.00 that was actually billed. This means that the amount applied to the plan deductible will be $60.00. The amount paid at the plan percentage is based on the lower amount of $60.00.

Whether the provider is in network or out of network will determine what impact this lower-than-billed reimbursement will have on the patient's wallet and the provider's revenue.

MEDICARE FEE SCHEDULE

Medicare is one of the few health carriers that provide access to the actual allowed amounts for the services that a provider will render to a patient. The source for this information is the Medicare Fee Schedule.

What is a Medicare Fee Schedule?

A Medicare Fee Schedule is a comprehensive list of CPT-4/HCPCS codes along with their corresponding allowed amounts. These amounts are used to reimburse providers for services rendered to patients covered under traditional Medicare plans.

The Centers for Medicare and Medicaid Services (CMS) also publishes separate fee schedules for physicians, ambulance services, clinical laboratory services, as well as durable medical equipment, prosthetics, orthotics, and supplies.

The Information on a Medicare Fee Schedule

HCPCS CODE	MODIFIER	SHORT DESCRIPTION	PROC STAT	MAC LOCALITY	NON-FACILITY PRICE	FACILITY PRICE	NON FACILITY LIMITING CHARGE	FACILITY LIMITING CHARGE	CONV. FACT
99214		Office/outpatient visit est.	A	1120201	$102.63	$76.19	$112.13	$83.23	35.8043
99215		Office/outpatient visit est.	A	1120201	$138.49	$107.80	$151.30	$117.77	35.8043

Breakdown by Field

- **HCPCS Code** – the CPT-4/HCPCS code/s for the service.
- **Modifier** – modifiers that can be billed with that procedure code.
- **Short Description** – a short description of the HCPCS code.
- **Proc Stat** – if this procedure code is an active or inactive code.
- **Mac Locality** – this number corresponds to the location of the carrier responsible for claim payment. Some states may have more than one carrier location.
- **Non-Facility Price** – reimbursement amount for services performed in a provider's office.
- **Facility Price** – reimbursement amount for services performed in a hospital or Ambulatory Surgical Center (ASC).
- **Non-Facility Limiting Charge** –this is the maximum amount that a nonparticipating provider can bill a Medicare beneficiary.
- **Facility Limiting Charge** – this is the maximum amount that a nonparticipating provider facility can bill a Medicare beneficiary.
- **Conv Fact-** the conversion factor that is used to come up with the allowed amounts.

Looking at this example

For billing code 99214, carrier location 1120201, a provider (non-facility) will be paid $102.63. This represents the allowed amount only. The $102.63 will be subject to any applicable deductible and coinsurance amounts.

For a Medicare patient, whose deductible is met for the year, the plan will pay $82.10 ($102.63 x 80%). The patient or a secondary plan would be responsible for the remaining 20%.

The Medicare Fee Schedule also provides detailed information on surgical procedures. In addition to the surgical allowed amounts, you can obtain information on how the services that are incidental to the surgery may be paid.

For Example

- Which modifiers will be accepted for the procedure?
- Is coverage available for bi-lateral or multiple surgeries, same session?
- Whether assistant, co surgeons or team surgeons will be paid.
- What is the global follow up period?

So how is this data used?

You have a patient with a Medicare plan that is coming into the office for an exam, urinalysis and a chest x-ray. Using the correct CPT-4/HCPCS codes, you will access the Medicare fee schedule at www.cms.gov, determine the allowed amounts for each procedure and use this information to set your expectations, including:

- What level of reimbursement can be expected from Medicare?
- How much can you expect to collect from the patient before they leave the office?

- How much do you expect to write off?

More and more commercial health carriers are starting to use the CMS (Centers for Medicare and Medicaid Services) fee schedule, instead of UCR as a basis to determine what will be allowed on a billed claim.

The Medicare fee schedule is easy to access, comprehensive and it seems to be in line with some of the contracted rates used by some commercial health carriers.

A PDF/Excel version of the Medicare Fee Schedule is located at www.cms.gov

MEDICAID FEE SCHEDULE

Some state Medicaid carriers publish the "allowed amounts" for most of the services, treatment and supplies that healthcare providers perform. This information is provided on the Medicaid Fee Schedule.

So what is a Medicaid Fee Schedule?

A Medicaid Fee Schedule is a detailed list of CPT-4/HCPCS codes along with their corresponding allowed amounts. These amounts are used to pay providers for the service rendered to patients covered under Medicaid plans. The fee schedule also helps the health provider to understand what they can expect to be reimbursed and what portion they are required to adjust off the account. Medicaid prohibits collecting upfront or balance billing Medicaid patients.

Medicaid does not have a "standard" way to administer their plans. This means, don't expect that every state's Medicaid will operate the same:

- Every state has some discretion in the way that care is delivered, claims are processed and payments are made.
- Medicaid plans could range from a Fee for Service plan to a Managed Care plan.

- Plans could be administered by the state or they could use a commercial health carrier to handle all claim related issues, enrollments, and claim payments.

Reimbursement could also range greatly from one state to the next. For example, Medicaid reimbursement is higher in California than it is in Louisiana because the cost to live in California is more expensive. Cost of living is one of the many factors that are used to come up with this pricing data.

You can usually locate the Medicaid Fee Schedule online at the state website for patients with non-managed care plans that are administered through the state. You will have to visit the website for each state to pull their respective fee schedules.

You will not have access to the Fee schedule for Medicaid managed care plans that are administered by a commercial health insurance carrier because they do not publish or provide access to this information.

Medicaid Reimbursement

The Medicaid fee schedule contains data on hundreds of codes. The overall perception that Medicaid payments are always extremely low may not be the case for all states and all procedures. Some codes are priced lower in some states while in other states that same code could be priced higher.

Most Medicaid plans pay at 100% of allowed. So you may not find a huge reimbursement difference between a commercial PPO plan, for example, that pays 80% with deductible and a Medicaid plan that pays slightly lower reimbursement but pays at 100%.

For Example

Chris P. has a PPO plan that pays 80% of the in network allowed amount with no deductible. His recent visit of $200.00 will be reduced to $150.00 with $120.00 paid by the carrier and $30.00 paid by the patient.

$150.00 total paid/$50.00 adjustment

If Chris had Medicaid, using the same example, reimbursement may look like this.

Using the fee schedule:

- The $200.00 is reduced to $120.00.
- $120.00 is paid to provider.
- $80.00 is adjusted off.
- $0.00 is paid by patient.

The payment to the provider may be slightly lower, but the patient portion could be eliminated; making this easier on the patient.

Medicaid Fee Schedules are usually available online at the Medicaid State website.

EFT VS. PAPER CHECKS

As technology advances, the way that data is now delivered provides faster and easier access to information and payment.

Daily, it seems I receive an email asking me to go online to register for paperless billing. I can now receive online statements for my light, gas and even my car payments and all can be set up to pay automatically, every month, without even a thought from me. Also, most of us have our paychecks automatically deposited into our accounts with online access to the statement readily available for review.

Well, that is the premise of EFT payments- a totally paperless way to receive claim payments.

EFT Payments

Electronic Funds Transfer (EFT) is payment through an electronic transfer of money from one bank to another bank. A provider can enroll with a health insurance carrier to have all payments delivered straight to the provider's bank account, electronically. These payments will hit the bank real time. In most cases, daily deposits. With the electronic submission of claim payments, you may also have the ability to have the EOB/RA submitted electronically as well. No more paper checks to hassle with.

EFT is far superior to paper checks because they allow for:

- Faster access to the funds.
- Faster patient invoicing.
- Faster reconciliation of the account.
- Faster secondary billing.
- Faster appeal and disputes for incorrect payment.
- A more secure, HIPAA compliant, way to transmit data and payment.
- Lower overhead. You may be able to eliminate at least one paid person that handles the mail room function as there is no need to have someone open and distribute mail.

Since Medical Billers do far more than just bill claims, most of us are responsible for appeals and disputes, account reconciliation, payment posting and collections. So, the faster the access to data the better.

I deal with EFT payments daily and I would be remiss if I did not paint all sides of the picture. Electronic Funds transfers do have one negative. Sometimes, it is difficult to identify who the payment belongs to and this inability to identify can slow down payment posting. Normally, the payment is received electronically and, with the exception of the EFT number and carrier & provider information, you have no patient identifying information. You can go online, type in the EFT number and try to back into the patient's EOB/RA so you can reconcile the account or you can wait for the EOB/RA to arrive.

Paper Checks

I am sure that we will never be able to go totally paperless because some health carriers, especially the smaller ones, have been slow to embrace EFT payments. Paper checks have so many negatives compared to EFT payments, including:

- Someone has to be paid to pick up, open and distribute the mail.
- Someone has to physically drive to the bank to deposit the checks.
- It takes days for you to have access to the funds due to the period between the date the check was issued and the date the check is mailed.

Paper checks are the least secure, non HIPAA compliant way to transmit information. If someone steals the mail not only would it takes weeks for the check to be replaced, they will gain access to a patient's Protected Health Information (PHI).

WRITE OFFS/ADJUSTMENTS

Write off and adjustment refers to the portion of the billed charges that a **participating provider** is required to remove from a patient's account. In my opinion, write off and adjustment mean the same thing but depending on the carrier, these terms may differ.

Participating providers agree not to bill the patient for any amount that exceeds the allowed amount. This requirement is clearly stated in the contract that a provider signs upon enrollment to participate. This means that the patient is not responsible for paying this portion of the billed charges.

For Example

Bill has a PPO plan with 100% in network coverage, no deductible. While working on his car, he cuts his finger. He consults his plan's provider directory and locates a participating provider in his area who can see him right away. The cut is minor so it is cleaned and dressed. The claim is processed:

$585.00 is billed to his carrier.

$185.00 is considered to be over the contracted rate.

$400.00 is deemed to be the allowed amount.

$400.00 is paid to the provider

$185.00 is the write off amount

This does not mean that the patient is being given a discount. A discount, as it relates to health care charges, means that the provider has decided to give a special reduction to their fee. Any discount to a patient must result in that same discount being billed to the health carrier as well.

Using the same example:

The doctor decides to give Bill a new patient discount of 20%. This amount would be taken off of the top and the claim would reflect this.

$585.00 -20% =$117.00

$468.00 ($585.00-$117.00) would now be the total that is billed to the health carrier.

In a Nutshell

Providers that participate are prohibited from balance billing any amounts that are over the contracted rate for a service, supply or treatment. A write off or adjustment is usually determined by the health carrier and is the portion that the health carrier will not consider on a billed claim.

A write off/adjustment may be required for a lot of reasons, usually when it's:

- Over the contracted rate.
- Over the Medicare allowed.
- Over the Medicaid allowed.
- As a result of a failure to have a Medicare patient sign an ABN as required for some services.

The amount to be adjusted off is usually clearly noted on the EOB/Remittance Advice. A review of the EOB will help you to determine if an adjustment is warranted. If unsure, call the carrier to clarify how the claim was calculated so that you can dispute any claims paid not as expected.

This adjustment or write off will take place after the patient and health carrier have both paid their portion of the bill; yet a balance still remains. At this point, the adjustment will be applied to the account - resulting in a zero balance.

Commercial health insurance carriers do not publish contracted rates, making it difficult to know in advance, how claims may be paid. For common procedures, you can keep a cheat sheet, by health carrier, that lists all procedures with corresponding allowed amounts. Health carriers do make errors, this way you can make sure that all claims are paid correctly.

See the section on allowed amounts for a detailed explanation.

COLLECTING UPFRONT

Health plans are written with the expectation that a patient will pay some portion of the healthcare services that they receive. This means that before you can even get comfortable in the waiting room and pick up one of those old magazines, you will be asked to pull out that credit card.

Collecting upfront is critical to revenue management as it is very difficult to collect from a patient after they have left the office. Revenue management is all about cash flow and keeping your eye on all outstanding account receivables. It is not just about the money due from health insurance carriers but money due from patients as well.

The key to collecting upfront is to contact the health carrier, prior to the visit, to verify eligibility and benefits. You need to know:

- What portion of the plan deductible has not been met?
- What is the coinsurance amount?
- Any limits that may affect coverage.
- Is the service covered?
- Is the patient eligible?

Understanding what the carrier pays and the patient's responsibility helps you to set the expectations for payment. This is not always easy to figure out because pricing data is not easily accessible. What to charge upfront is sometimes a mystery, leaving patients to worry if they will get reimbursed if they pay more than the allowed amount.

Online access to EOB's/RA's can help a bit. You may be able to pull an old EOB/RA from one of the patient's past visits for a similar or same service that the patient is being seen for. This way you will know exactly how the claim was processed and what the patient's true upfront costs will be.

Most patients have no idea how health insurance really works. Taking the time to educate them about their particular plan gives them the chance to prepare, not just emotionally, but financially for each visit. Patients need to know what to expect when they reach the office. The expectation of payment should be passed on when the patient is called to confirm the appointment. It is frustrating for patients to reach the office with little or no expectation of payment and be asked to pay before they can even see the doctor.

I think that most of us are still not totally comfortable with asking patients to pay upfront, especially when we know that this may create a hardship for them but this is a plan expectation and under some plans, like Medicare for one, this is a plan requirement.

Medicare does not allow a provider to waive copays, deductibles or coinsurance amounts unless due to hardship. Even in hardship cases, Medicare requires that you make 3 attempts to collect before you can write it off as a bad debt.

Bottom line, contact the health carrier, set your expectations for payment and always collect from the patient before they leave the office.

EXPLANATION OF BENEFITS/REMITTANCE ADVICE

It seems to me that I've spent my life either looking for EOB's/RA's, waiting for EOB's/RA's to arrive, reviewing EOB's/RA's or disputing EOB's/RA's.

Review all EOB's as soon as they come in. More and more plans are moving toward 60 days from the date of the EOB to dispute a claim. Do not lose the ability to get correct payment.

In this business, EOB/RA's provide that sought after information that tells you everything you need to know about a claim. In fact, they tell more than just how a claim was processed; they also tell you:

- That you are doing a great job because the claim was processed with no delays, no hold ups, no problems – just payment.
- That you missed something critical that was needed to move the claim through. This way you can learn from it, note it for future claims and not repeat the mistake.
- That something is changing. A service, treatment or supply that before breezed through claim processing with no problem is now being scrutinized, held, or denied by the health carrier. This "heads up" gives you the chance to keep your eye on this issue to see how it will affect future

payments. Maybe you will go to the carrier website to see if the criterion for coverage has changed or if a modifier is now required, implement more upfront testing or documentation to support your need, or maybe just change your internal procedures.

For example

In my business, it is not uncommon for our patients to receive more than one of the same items. In reviewing an EOB/RA from a particular carrier, I discovered that if more than one item was billed, only one was being paid. So I called the health carrier who informed me about the "day limit." They now will pay for only one of the same items, per day. This advanced warning allowed us to change the way we handled items to this carrier before any more claims were denied.

So what is an EOB/RA?

An EOB (Explanation of Benefits) or RA (Remittance Advice) is a statement prepared by the insurance carrier that explains how the claim was processed. In my opinion, EOB and RA mean basically the same thing but, depending on the health carrier, the term may differ.

The EOB/RA provides information about the final adjudication of the claim, including:

- Payments
- Allowed amounts
- Deductibles
- Co-pays
- Adjustments
- Not covered amounts
- Deductible and Out of pocket amounts that are met to date

- Denials
- Refunds
- Appeal/Dispute processes
- Various status codes that further explain how a claim was processed

The EOB/RA should be reviewed thoroughly as it tells you what the next step should be on that claim, including:

- If you need to submit additional information on the claim.
- If the balance is due from the patient.
- If the secondary carrier needs to be billed.
- If the balance is adjusted off.
- If you need to file an appeal or dispute (claim underpaid or paid incorrectly).
- If you need to contact the patient because they need to provide additional information.
- If a claim paid as expected and you need to close the account.

EOB's are excellent sources of data on allowed amounts. I keep a cheat sheet of my most common codes with the allowed amounts by carrier. This helps me to have some idea what will be allowed so I know what to collect upfront. This will not be exact, as reimbursement will differ, but this will get you fairly close.

Please note that an EOB will be issued for paid as well as zero paid claims.

For example

A claim for $150.00 is billed to the health carrier; $125.00 for the office visit and $25.00 for a flu shot. The

$125.00 is applied to the plan deductible and the $25.00 is not covered under the plan.

Even though no payment was made, the process of review and reconciliation is the same.

You may need to bill a secondary plan, invoice the patient, or maybe review the plan to see if, as an in network provider, the deductible should not have applied.

Please refer to Chapter Eight under "How To Read an EOB/RA" for more information.

Difficult claim? I suggest making a cheat sheet noting any modifiers or special handling that was needed to get this claim to payment.

APPEALS/DISPUTES

When pre-authorization is denied or the claim is not paid as expected, the appeal/dispute process begins. To me, the words appeal and dispute mean the same thing but depending on the health carrier, the terminology and the process may differ.

All insurance carriers represent themselves as providing necessary medical care to plan holders, yet oftentimes we must go to extraordinary lengths to get them to uphold their end of the deal.

Every insurance carrier has some type of dispute/appeal process and every provider should exercise their right to get reimbursed, as expected, and in most cases, as promised.

So what is an appeal/dispute?

Basically, this means to disagree with how a benefit/coverage was applied or a payment/process was handled and asking the health carrier to make the appropriate corrections.

When should a claim be appealed/disputed?

In my opinion EVERY CLAIM that was not processed as expected should be disputed. This applies to, not only providers, but patients as well.

Not sure what to say on appeal?

Just stick to the basics

- How was the claim handled or paid.
- Why you believe an error has occurred.
- How you expect them to fix it.

Real World Example

Cindy J. has a Medicare HMO plan. She received treatment that is normally covered by traditional Medicare; yet it was denied by the Medicare HMO plan as "not covered under her plan." Cindy is upset that a service she considers "necessary" is not covered so she contacted me to help. I contact the health carrier who continues to state that the service is not covered. I review the back of the EOB for the correct appeal procedures and I submit my appeal letter on the patient's behalf. My appeal letter is simple, just the facts:

1. The carrier denied the claim.
2. The carrier had no basis to deny because Medicare managed care plans are required to provide the same or better level of coverage than traditional Medicare. ***Not less coverage.***
3. We expect the claim to be reprocessed.
4. I attach a copy of the Medicare fee schedule that supports the fact that this service is covered.

Final outcome: The claim is reprocessed by the health carrier.

My Thoughts

This is where I think the true value of outsourcing or having an Insurance Specialist on staff lies.

First - The Insurance Specialist will know how they expected the claim to be reimbursed and if that expectation is not met, they will know how the resolution process should begin.

Second- The Insurance Specialist will understand the basis of the denial or underpayment.

Third - The Insurance Specialist will know if the "dispute" can be handled by a call to the carrier or by a formal complaint.

Example: The carrier paid the claim out of network but it should have been paid in network. One call to the carrier can resolve this fairly easily.

Fourth - The Insurance Specialist will put procedures in place to ensure that if an error occurred due to internal miscommunication, billing errors or training issues, it will not be repeated.

Fifth - If a formal appeal/dispute is required, the Insurance Specialist will determine the correct way this should be handled. Some carriers require a completed appeal form with a signed permission slip from the plan holder while others allow you to put your dispute in writing and fax it over. Some carriers have an Appeal/Dispute Department while others say mail the dispute to attention "Claims."

The back of the EOB usually will provide the steps to handling an appeal/dispute. You can also check the health carrier's website.

For more detailed information, please visit Chapter Eight and view the article on "How to Appeal a Claim."

REVENUE MANAGEMENT

We have mentioned the word ***reimbursement*** numerous times on the pages of this guide. Our goal was to help you understand that when it is all said and done, everything we do all comes down to that one word. Steady, consistent reimbursement is critical to effective revenue management.

So what is Revenue Management?

Revenue management is this new buzz word, but really it is not new to anyone whose primary responsibility is to manage billing and the resulting open account receivables.

To me, simplistically, Revenue Management is all about keeping your eye on all aspects of a provider's practice to make sure that there is a steady flow of new patients and a steady flow of reimbursement and that claims are being billed correctly and timely and aging open accounts are minimal. This may mean improving communication, streamlining processes, managing expenses or a combination of all three.

To me, the process has to work like a like a chain, starting and never ending, unbroken with no kinks.

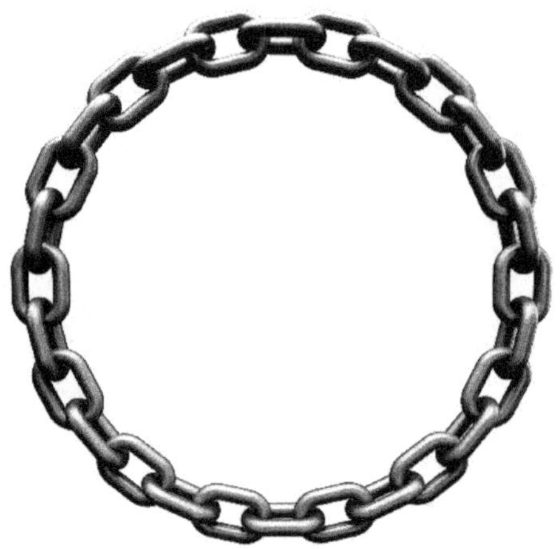

Services are performed - claims are billed - claims are paid resulting in cash flow - overhead expenses, salaries, and insurances are paid - practice is profitable - all processes are monitored - start over.

The providers, front office staff and medical billers are the people most responsible for keeping that chain flowing and unbroken. Failure to do any of the following may result in a disruption to one or more parts of the chain, creating less than expected cash flow resulting in less income needed to pay salaries and overhead, leading to poor revenue management. Some examples of poor revenue management include:

- Not collecting upfront.
- Not verifying benefits and eligibility.
- Not billing claims correctly
- Not billing claims timely.
- Not following up on all unpaid, aging claims, timely.
- Not appealing all incorrect payments, timely.
- Not keeping accurate payer information.
- Not communicating any problems that may result in loss of income.

As a medical biller, you have the responsibility of not only billing a claim, but of also having the knowledge that is needed to get that claim reimbursed. Partner a good understanding of health insurance processes with a good understanding of medical billing and coding and you have the fierce combination needed to master revenue management.

I have seen both sides of the process, I have worked for health insurance carriers scrutinizing claims that are submitted by health providers and I have also billed claims to health carriers. I believe that revenue management is tougher in this industry because reimbursement is so hard to predict. But I truly believe patients are the heart of this business.

In some businesses you can sell more or increase pricing as a way to improve the bottom line. In some businesses you can even use fewer humans and rely more on call centers and automated systems to help control costs. But this simply won't do in the health insurance business. We are driven by contracted rates and fee schedules and a "pick me from the directory" approach to capturing more patients but we are committed to providing patients with good care and live interaction.

Revenue management is critical to the success of any good practice but if you lack the resources internally, I believe that outsourcing the medical billing function may be the solution. Outsourcing to the right medical billers will have a positive impact on the bottom line.

The right people:

- Truly know and understand this business.
- Know how to navigate through the process.
- Are keeping an eye on the bottom line because that is how they get paid.
- Are keeping their eye on the numerous changes that affect reimbursement.

CHAPTER SEVEN TEST

Directions: Using what you have learned in Chapter Seven, match the correct term to the appropriate definition.

A	Contracted rate		The amount the provider is required to adjust off a patient's account.
B	UCR		The electronic transfer of claim payments.
C	Allowed amount		A statement that shows how a claim was processed.
D	Fee schedule		Reimbursement rate that is agreed to, by contract, between a participating provider and the health carrier.
E	EFT		Contacting the health carrier to dispute the way a claim was processed.
F	Write off		The usual or average charge for a service, treatment or supply.
G	EOB		The portion of the billed charges that are covered by the plan.
H	Appeal		The process of keeping ones eye on all aspects of a provider's practice to ensure that it is profitable.
I	Revenue Management		A list of the allowed amounts for each valid CPT code.

8 HOW TO

Chapter Overview - Failure to miss any step in the claims process could result in payment that is less than expected. In this section, we show you how to navigate the day-to-day processes that are critical to ensuring the best medical and financial outcome.

This Chapter Includes:

HOW TO SUBMIT FOR REFERRAL

A Medical Biller could have a wide range of duties and responsibilities besides just billing claims. They may be expected to handle appeals and disputes, follow up on unpaid claims, review EOB's, post payments, reconcile accounts and handle collections.

If the medical biller works in a medical provider's office, those duties may include a host of other frontend and backend tasks, including the need to ***facilitate a referral.***

A referral grants "permission" for patients with managed care plans to seek services or specialty care that either, cannot be provided by the Primary Care Physician, or cannot be provided in network.

Some plan types, like PPO plans for one, do not require a patient to obtain a referral. PPO plan members can simply call any provider that they wish to see, schedule an appointment and pay the required out of pocket costs. But other plan types are way more restrictive. HMO and EPO plans are two types where a referral is mandatory or the claim will be denied.

The Primary Care Physician's office is responsible for facilitating a referral on a patient's behalf. A patient cannot facilitate their own referral request nor can they bypass this process; unless they plan to pay out of pocket.

The Primary Care Physician will determine if the request is warranted based on medical necessity. If approved, the PCP will provide a copy of the referral for the patient to take with them during their initial visit with the out-of-network provider or specialist.

How are referrals handled?

Since the PCP is usually the treating doctor, they may have already recognized the need to elevate care to the next level so they may have already started the referral process. But in some situations, such as a new patient being seen for the first time, a patient that has not been seen for a while, a patient already being seen by a specialist but requiring care by another specialist or a patient that requests to be seen by a provider that is out of network, the need to obtain a referral in advance is mandatory.

Bottom line, the PCP is responsible for approving all care in advance, so you must start with them. Some providers have a Referral Department that will handle the paperwork part of this once the PCP grants approval. In order to get the referral started you will need to:

- Pull all supporting documentation, including test results, patient history and physicals. Gather anything that supports why the referral should be granted.
- Have the Primary Care Physician review the file and all pertinent information to confirm that a referral is medically necessary. Most providers have a list of providers of all specialties that they refer to.
- Once the PCP has granted approval, the paperwork must be completed so that a record of referral is on file. This will ensure that all claims will be paid correctly.
- Make sure the PCP is aware of any health issues that may affect the urgency of the request.

The entire process may take a week or so to complete, but if medically warranted, the request will be approved.

A referral may be denied if:

- The proposed care can be provided in network.
- The proposed care is deemed not medically necessary.
- There is not enough information to support coverage.

The denial can be appealed by providing the additional support that is needed to move this to approval.

Most referrals have a start and end date. Please make sure that the visit falls within those parameters or the claim will be denied.

HOW TO SUBMIT FOR PREAPPROVAL

A Medical Biller could have a wide scope of duties and responsibilities. Besides billing claims, you may also be required to handle appeals and disputes, follow up on all open claim accounts, post payments, reconcile accounts and handle collections. And if you happen to work in a medical provider's office, those duties may include a host of other frontend and backend tasks which may include the need to ***facilitate a preapproval request.***

For patients covered under a managed care plan, the need to follow the rules of the plan is critical to the level of reimbursement that one can expect.

Failure to secure preapproval, in advance, may result in a reduced payment or denial of the claim.

The terms pre-authorization and pre-approval are used interchangeably and, depending on the carrier, may mean the same.

Pre-approval is simply the health carrier's assurance that the service(s) in question is/are deemed to be medically necessary, and appropriate, based on the patient's current condition.

For example, a chest x-ray may not be appropriate for a patient with a broken leg.

Every pre-approval letter will include a disclaimer by the health carrier that states that a preapproval is not a guarantee of payment. This is because the preapproval process ***does not*** normally include a review of the patient's current benefit plan. Meaning, it is possible that you can be granted pre-approval for a service or supply and the claim end up being denied because the service is not covered under the patient's plan.

The Preapproval Process Needs Two Steps:

1. Call the health insurance carrier to obtain eligibility and benefits. You may need to speak to a Customer Service Representative (CSR) directly to inquire if a particular service or supply is covered and if any plan or frequency limits exist that may affect payment. The CSR can also provide the number of the Utilization Review (UR) Department as well as the appropriate billing addresses.

If you provide the CSR with the CPT-4/HCPCS code for a particular treatment service or supply they can look them up for you to confirm coverage and even allowed amounts.

---

2. Contact the UR Department to facilitate pre-approval. The first question should always be, does this service or supply require pre-approval? You may find that some services under a certain dollar amount or some very common procedures do not require pre-approval. If pre-approval is required, you may be directed online to download and complete a PA form. They may also take the full information over the phone.

Be prepared to provide all or some of the following:

- Patient's insurance ID, home address and contact info.
- Relationship to the plan holder.
- Provider name, address, NPI/Tax ID numbers and specialty.

- ICD-10 codes.
- CPT-4/HCPCS codes.
- Duration of treatment.
- Expected date of treatment.
- History and Physical, test results and any other supporting documentation that can support the need for the service.

Please make the UR Department aware of any special circumstance or unusual factors that may affect the process. You should also let the UR nurse know if the patient's condition requires expedited review and decision.

The case will be reviewed and a coverage decision granted in about 1-15 days, on average, depending on the carrier, procedure and urgency. Be sure to update the insurance carrier if the patient's condition changes and be sure to follow up within a reasonable time.

Make sure you have the pre-approval in writing, not just an authorization number on your voicemail, this way you have the support needed to dispute any incorrect payments.

The UR Department is normally a completely separate internal department or in some cases an outside company that has been contracted with a health insurance carrier to provide UR support. Because of this, you may notice a big disconnect between the Claims and UR Departments. Meaning, the UR Department may issue an approval but the Claims Department may not have that approval on file which could result in an incorrect claim payment. Because of this, make sure that all claims are paid correctly.

HOW TO APPEAL MEDICARE

Out of all of my many years in this industry, I can count the number of times, on one hand, that I have appealed a Medicare claim. Nevertheless, Medicare provides comprehensive information on their website (www.cms.gov) on everything from education and training to coverage policies and fee schedules. I use this site as my go to place when I am trying to figure out what I need to do to ensure that a Medicare claim will get paid.

But no amount of preparation guarantees that an error will not occur. If you believe that a Medicare claim has been processed incorrectly or has been denied in error, you have the right to initiate an appeal. Medicare has a 4 level appeal process.

FIRST LEVEL OF APPEAL:

Redetermination by a Medicare Contractor

APPEAL LEVEL:
REDETERMINATION

TIME LIMIT FOR FILING REQUEST:

60 days from when the claim was processed incorrectly.

MONETARY THRESHOLD TO BE MET:

None

Complete a CMS-20027 form and attach any and all documentation that supports the reason why the claim should be reprocessed. This request must be sent to the same Medicare carrier that initially processed the claim. You will be advised of the written decision in a Medicare Redetermination Notice (MRN) within 60 days.

SECOND LEVEL OF APPEAL:

Reconsideration by a Qualified Independent Contractor

If the first level appeal is upheld, you have the option to go to a second level appeal. Using a CMS-20033 form, a copy of the MRN letter and all supporting documentation; including the reason you disagree with the decision and feel the claim should be reprocessed. The form and all supporting documents will be sent to the Qualified Independent Contractor (QIC) for the appropriate jurisdiction. The QIC will send written decision within 60 days.

APPEAL LEVEL:
RECONSIDERATION

TIME LIMIT FOR FILING REQUEST:

60 days from the date of receipt of the Redetermination Decision.

MONETARY THRESHOLD TO BE MET:

None

Original Medicare (Fee-For-Service) Qualified Independent Contractors

The following is a list of the QICs and the jurisdictions that they serve:

Part A East Jurisdiction:	Maximus, Inc.
Part A West Jurisdiction:	C2C Solutions, Inc.
Part B North Jurisdiction:	C2C Solutions, Inc.
Part B South Jurisdiction:	C2C Solutions, Inc.
DME Jurisdiction:	C2C Solutions, Inc.

THIRD LEVEL OF APPEAL:

Hearing by an Administrative Law Judge

APPEAL LEVEL:
ADMINISTRATIVE LAW JUDGE (ALJ)

TIME LIMIT FOR FILING REQUEST:

60 days from the date of receipt of the Reconsideration Decision.

MONETARY THRESHOLD TO BE MET:

Visit www.cms.gov for current info

If the second appeal is also upheld, you have the option of a third level appeal by an Administrative Law Judge (ALJ). The amount in question must meet the threshold. The Reconsideration notice of decision will have instructions on how to initiate a third level appeal using a CMS-20034 form. ALJ hearings are usually held by video-teleconference (VTC) or by telephone, but you can ask for an in-person hearing. The ALJH will provide a decision within 90 days.

FOURTH LEVEL OF APPEAL:

Review by the Medicare Appeal Council

If the third level of appeal is also upheld, you have one final option – review by the Medicare Appeal Council. The ALJ decision letter will have instructions on how to file this final appeal. A written decision will be given within 90 days.

<u>APPEAL LEVEL:</u>
DEPARTMENTAL APPEALS BOARD (DAB) REVIEW/APPEALS COUNCIL

<u>TIME LIMIT FOR FILING REQUEST:</u>

60 days from the date of receipt of the ALJ Hearing Decision.

<u>MONETARY THRESHOLD TO BE MET:</u>

None

Note: If all four Medicare appeals fail, you may have the option of going above Medicare by requesting a Federal Court Review. Visit www.cms.gov for details on this process.

The appeal process is not just for providers. A patient can open their own appeal if they disagree with the way that Medicare processed a claim.

Real World Example

A patient ordered a promotional item that was cute and fun and matched the outfit she was wearing on vacation, but it clearly was not a medically necessary item. Because it was sold at the same place where she purchased other medically necessary supplies, she felt that it should be covered.

She signed an ABN, paid the $36.00 in costs and requested that the claim be billed to Medicare. The claim was billed and it was denied as expected.

She is now on the 4th level of appeal and, in spite of the repeated denials, she has vowed to appeal this claim to the end. Just because a claim is appealed, does not mean that the original denial will be overturned. But the process is in place to give everyone that right to be heard.

Go to the www.cms.gov for additional details on this process.

HOW TO APPEAL MEDICAID

I work with Medicaid in just about every state so I know firsthand that the way that Medicaid plans can be administered could add a whole different level of complexity to both the billing and appeals processes. For instance:

- Traditional Medicaid plans are normally administered by each state, meaning that claims are billed to and paid by the state. Any inquiries will be directed to the particular state where the patient has coverage.
- Managed care plans are usually administered by commercial health insurance carriers. This means you would have to call the health carrier directly, not the state Medicaid, to obtain plan, payment or processing information.
- Every Medicaid carrier has some say over how they administer Medicaid plans, so the process for handling a Medicaid claim could differ greatly by state.

The path to appealing or disputing a Medicaid claim is not always cut and dry, so you have to make sure you are confident that all front end processes are in place. Make sure you have a copy of the front and back of the patient's ID card and that you call the health carrier to confirm eligibility, benefits, who administers the plan and where claims should be filed.

The most common reasons for appeal are:

- Eligibility issues
- Authorization issues
- Underpayment or incorrect payments
- Plan confusion because the patient failed to disclose that they switched from one plan type to another.

How to Handle the Appeal

If you discover that a Medicaid claim has been paid incorrectly or denied in error, the back of the EOB will provide information on how to start the appeal or dispute process.

Always start with a call to the health carrier. This is the fastest and easiest way to resolve an issue. If a billing error exists, the carrier will be able to walk you through the correction process so you can rebill the claim.

The appeal process will usually require that you complete some type of appeal form. This form can normally be found online at the state Medicaid, or the commercial carrier's websites. You will need to include any and all pertinent documentation, including:

- Claim copy (if needed).
- The RA/EOB.
- Treatment authorization request.
- Service authorization request.
- Invoice (if needed).
- Any other documents that supports your reason for appeal.

Make sure you clearly state the reason for appeal and stick to the facts. Also include how you wish to have this issue resolved. Mail, fax, or upload your appeal as instructed. The appeal will normally be acknowledged within 10-15 days from receipt, with a decision in about 45 days.

The key is to:

- Always appeal all incorrect payments.
- Do your research. Make sure you understand the basis for appeal, what information should accompany the appeal and how to start the appeal process, i.e. online form, call to carrier, etc.
- Keep a cheat sheet of the process so you can easily duplicate it.
- Make sure that you take the time to get clear about a patient's coverage before service is rendered. Also, always make sure that you verify eligibility frequently as Medicaid coverage could change month to month.

Medicaid prohibits balance billing to Medicaid patients so failure to handle everything correctly on the front end could be costly if a claim is not paid.

Note: This is merely a guide to the process; please check the website of the state Medicaid carrier to obtain the specific instructions on how to handle an appeal for the state in question.

HOW TO APPEAL A COMMERCIAL CLAIM

On a daily basis, I find the need to appeal or dispute a claim that has been incorrectly paid by commercial health insurance carriers. I am not saying that they are always at fault, because errors occur on both sides, but the need to dispute or appeal a claim is all part of the job.

The key to appealing to a commercial health insurance carrier is to:

First - Do your homework. Make sure that the error is in fact the fault of the health carrier and not because you failed to obtain the correct information upfront or you failed to obtain a needed referral or preapproval.

Second - Do not back down until the issue is resolved. When you call a health insurance carrier, the experience of the Claim Processor could vary greatly. There are no schools, that I know of, that teach claim processing. Most are taught on the job, they could have years of experience or they could have just recently come out of training. The ability to resolve your issue, effectively, will vary greatly, so insist on speaking to a supervisor if are unable to resolve the issue to your satisfaction.

Third - Before you place the call to the carrier have all of your ducks in a row. Make sure you have everything you need to resolve the issue without having to call back.

You should have:

- Patient information
- Health plan information
- Carrier contact information
- Service dates and amount
- What error has occurred
- Copy of the EOB or denial letter

Step One

Explain the error and request a correction. Clearly state the reasons you believe the claim was paid incorrectly and stick to the facts. Also, tell the CSR how you think the issue should be resolved. If the CSR tells you that an online form is required, make sure to get the form number and where the form can be located online. Mail, fax, or upload your appeal as instructed. The appeal will normally be acknowledged within 10-15 days from receipt, with a decision in about 45 days.

If the CSR tells you that they "will have the claim sent back for correction," make sure you thoroughly document the call, including when you can expect to receive payment, the name of the person you spoke with and the reference number of the call. You are going to thank me for this tip when you have to call the carrier back about this same issue. ***Calendar this to make sure this payment arrives as expected.***

If the call to the carrier fails to get the claim reprocessed, move to step two.

Step Two

Health carriers are required to provide information on how to appeal a claim on all EOB's - the process will vary greatly based on the health insurance carrier.

Some health carriers simply request a letter detailing the reason that you feel the claim was not paid correctly while others may have a detailed process including a signed release from the patient. Others will not allow the provider to initiate an appeal, only the patient. Review the EOB for directions and contact the patient to enlist their help in getting the issue resolved.

After numerous unsuccessful attempts to resolve the issue. The patient will have the option of contacting either the Department of Insurance, if the plan is fully insured, or the Department of Labor if the plan is self-funded.

HOW TO VERIFY BENEFITS

Verifying benefits is the process of contacting the patient's insurance company to confirm that valid eligibility is on file and to obtain an overview of the patient's plan. The purpose being to:

- Understand how the visit may ultimately be paid.
- Determine how much the patient will have to pay up front for the visit.
- Determine if any referral, pre-authorization, pre-determination or pre-certification procedures must be handled prior to the visit.
- Determine if any plan benefits or limitations are in place that may affect the visit.
- Make sure that the patient is eligible under the plan.

Write down your expectations for payment, this way whoever posts the payments or makes reconciliations on the account will key into any payments that are not as expected.

Do not trust that a patient is still eligible for coverage or that a health care plan or insurance carrier has not changed. Patients have a tendency to ignore correspondence from health insurance carriers so they may not have the most accurate information or they may be confused about which plan they actually have.

For example, Medicare patients will insist that they have Medicare but they may have a managed care plan that is administered by a commercial carrier. Take the time to verify eligibility and benefits. Since eligibility could change monthly, especially for Medicaid patients, you may need to re-verify eligibility every month for some patients.

The Process

Before you call the health carrier, you will need several pieces of information. I suggest that you get a copy of the front and back of the patient's identification card. You will also need:

- The plan holder's name (the person who actually holds the insurance) and date of birth
- Their ID number
- Insurance carrier's telephone number
- Provider ID numbers - NPI or Tax ID or the Contract ID number
- Your name and call back number

It is important that you use an Insurance Verification Form of some sort; as they provide a "script" for you to follow and assures that nothing will be forgotten. Also, organize your time for different patients that have the same insurance companies by making these calls together.

Fill out the verification form as you go and make the completed form a part of the patient's record. Customer Service Reps have been known to provide erroneous information. You must have an accurate record just in case problems arise.

When you verify eligibility for out of network Providers, ask the carrier how the out of network claims will be reimbursed.

Most insurance carriers will dispatch you into the automated system for benefits and eligibility and provider mailing addresses. In the automated system, you can listen to the benefits or have them faxed over. I tend to listen first and then have them faxed over for my records.

You Need to Verify:

1. That the patient is currently eligible.
2. The effective date of coverage.
3. Type of plan PPO, HMO, POS, etc. Remember, different plans have different rules. An HMO plan may require a valid referral be in place or may provide no out of network benefits. For PPO, POS or EPO plans you may need to determine if the provider is in-network to ensure the maximum level of reimbursement.
4. The name of the Primary Care Physician (if applicable). The PCP's office will help facilitate any needed referrals and authorizations.
5. Benefits, including deductibles, copays and the reimbursement levels. This way you will know which portion of the bill the patient will be responsible for so that this amount can be collected up front. Always get benefits for the type of service that is to be performed. This will ensure that you are provided with the benefits and limitations that may apply to that service.
6. The correct mailing address for claims. Most insurance carriers have numerous addresses make sure you have the address to mail claims.

Keep in mind that the automated system can only go so far. It is designed to provide just the basics so don't hesitate to speak with a live person if you need to.

A live Customer Service Rep can answer the following:

1. Does the plan have any pre-certification, prior-authorization, pre-determination or referral requirements for the service that is to be rendered to the patient?
2. What is the phone number of the UR Department?
3. What is the "standard" processing time and how long before a claim is scanned into the system? Carriers can normally tell you after a week or so if they, at least, have your unprocessed claim on file.
4. What is the timely filing period?
5. What is the EDI submitter number for submitting claims electronically?

Remember that a Customer Service Rep is simply a messenger. Their role is to provide information on the plan, as written. They did not write the plan, nor do they have the authority to change it. This does not mean that you should simply accept poor service or incorrect or confusing information. If you have issues that need to be resolved, request to speak to a supervisor or manager since they would be better able to remedy the problem.

U/R Review

If preapproval, predetermination or precertification is required, you will be transferred over or provided the phone number for the U/R Department so that you can facilitate preapproval. The U/R Department can provide you with the list of documentation that will be needed to facilitate the request. For more information, refer to Chapter Eight, "How to Submit for Preapproval."

Always document this conversation thoroughly, including date of the call, the person that you spoke with and the call reference number.

More and more carriers are using the Medicare Fee Schedule instead of Usual Customary and Reasonable (UCR). The Medicare Fee Schedule is available online and it lists the fees for most procedures. This way you have some idea what to collect while the patient is still in the office.

HOW TO READ A SUMMARY PLAN DESCRIPTION

Upon enrollment in a health plan, the plan member is provided access to the booklet which describes the benefits and limits of the plan. This booklet may be referred to by numerous different terms including a Certificate of Coverage, Benefit Booklet, Summary Plan Description, Health Plan Document or even a Policy.

The Benefits Book may be available online at the health carrier's website or the plan member can request a copy from their Human Resource Department.

This booklet is simply a guide to everything you ever wanted to know about a health plan; from what is covered, what is not covered and everything in between.

***Insurance Carriers will refer to the SPD as a means to*:**

- Document the agreed upon terms and provisions of the plan.
- Understand and communicate the provisions of the plan.
- Adjudicate all claims in accordance with the provisions of the plan.

Patients will refer to the SPD as a means to:

- Understand how they should access care.
- Determine how to enroll dependents.
- Understand their rights when employment terminates.

Providers will refer to the SPD as a means to:

- Understand benefits of the plan so that the patient can be advised, upfront, of any financial liability.
- Understand the rules of the plan.
- Make sure that the insurance carrier is administrating the plan as written and that any gray areas can be clarified without penalty to the patient or the provider.

Reimbursement Specialists/Billers will refer to the SPD as a means to:

- Understand how to appeal all denied or incorrect payments.
- Challenge a provision or benefit that may not be administered as written or may be unclear.

This benefit booklet contains a lot of information including the:

Plan Summary

(A summary of the benefits and amounts)

Deductibles- The amount that you will have to pay before the plan starts to reimburse. Please note that the plan deductible is not paid to the insurance carrier. They will automatically subtract the deductible from the first claims received from each patient. They will continue to take the deducible until it is met in full.

Coinsurance level- The percentage that the plan will pay all covered charges at.

Out of pocket maximum - The maximum amount of covered charges that you will have to pay out of your pocket before the plan starts to pay at 100%.

Co-payment amount - The amount that you will have to pay out of your pocket per visit.

General benefits - How the plan will reimburse for a host of different types of services, including but not limited to, hospital and doctor's services, routine or well child care, mental/nervous and substance abuse care, chiropractic, physical therapy, ambulance, durable medical equipment and skilled or private duty nursing.

Benefit limitations/maximum - The maximum that a plan will pay for a particular benefit.

Lifetime Maximums - The maximum that the plan will pay in a person's lifetime.

Benefit Section

(Detailed provisions of the plan)

- ***Pre-admission/pre-certification requirements*** - This outlines what requirements are in place in the event you are hospitalized. Most plans require that you call a specific number to obtain "approval" for the hospital stay before you are confined. In the event of an emergency, you are normally given 24 hours to call.
- ***Preventative care*** - Outlines the benefits that may be available for preventative care including well child, vision, hearing and special woman's services.
- ***Major Medical*** - Explains in more detail, coverage periods, deductibles, coinsurance etc.
- ***Covered expenses*** - Details the plan's position on numerous services from allergy tests to organ transplants.

- ***Exclusions and limitations*** **-** A bullet by bullet list of all the services that are not covered under the plan.
- ***Claim procedures*** - Details the claim filing procedures (in network and out of network) and your appeal rights should you disagree with the insurance company's handling of a claim.
- ***Dental section*** **-** Details the covered and excluded dental services.
- ***Pharmacy*** - Details how medications will be covered. Most plans have a list of drugs called a formulary that are covered but they may have different levels of reimbursement.
- ***Vision section*** **-** Details about the covered and excluded vision service.

Administration Section

(How the plan will handle situations.)

Eligibility

- Who is eligible for coverage under the plan?
- When would you become eligible for coverage?
- Who are eligible dependents under the plan?
- How late enrollees are handled? (Members who do not take the plan when offered but try to join later.)

Termination

- When coverage terminates.
- Extension of benefits.
- Certificate of credible coverage information- A certificate that can be provided to your next insurance carrier as proof of coverage so that preexisting periods can be minimized or eliminated.

- COBRA – Provides for extension of the existing coverage.
- Family Medical Leave Act- Provides for up to 12 weeks of unpaid leave for certain reasons without the loss of the job.

USCRP **-** Uniformed Service Continuation and Reinstatement Provision- allows for continuation of coverage to and reinstatement of coverage for persons in the military.

COB **-** Coordination of Benefit (COB)- How claims will be paid and who pays first when you have two or more insurance plans.

Subrogation **-** Provides for the plan to recover the money that it had paid out on claims related to an illness or injury that is the caused by a third party.

I know people who will buy a toaster or a juicer or even a car and read the manual cover to cover yet they refuse to touch their benefit booklet. Don't expect that a patient will know or have any idea how to access care or what is covered. When in doubt, ask the patient to provide a copy of the SPD for review.

HOW TO READ AN EXPLANATION OF BENEFIT/REMITTANCE ADVICE

Medical Billers will spend a great deal of time reviewing EOB's. An EOB, or Remittance Advice (RA), is the statement from the health carrier that details exactly how the claim was processed. The EOB should provide both balance and closure meaning that it should provide a clear picture of how every dime of the billed claim was handled.

Depending on the scope of the job, a Medical Biller may not just bill claims; they also may be expected to be an Insurance Specialist. Insurance Specialists understand all aspects of health insurance and can almost predict how a claim will be processed.

Setting expectations and meeting those expectations is part of the job that we do.

Before I review an EOB, I usually review the patient's file to remind myself of what the expectations were for the claim. If the claim did not process as expected, ***I need to know why.***

Review all EOB's as soon as they come in. More and more plans are moving toward 60 days from the date of the EOB to dispute a claim. Do not lose the ability to get correct payment.

How to read An EOB

Because health insurance carriers cram so much information into an EOB/RA you should:

- Prepare yourself first. You may need a calculator and access to the remittance codes/definitions that are located at www.wpc-edi.com. WPC is Washington Publishing Company and they publish a series of codes that are standardly used by a lot of different health insurance carriers.
- Realize that EOB's do not always make sense. Health carriers use a series of codes to try to explain how a claim was processed. Hence, the reason why you may need a calculator and the coding information. Sometimes the codes and their meanings are located directly on the EOB and sometimes you are provided only the code and you have to go to the WPC website to get the meaning.
- Go over the EOB line by line. An EOB should provide total clarity on how the claim was handled; no mysteries. Every code and charge that was billed should be accounted for. If you are unable to resolve a discrepancy, call the carrier for help.

EOB Example

Refer to the example below of how a standard EOB may look and what data they provide.

How to read an Explanation of Benefit Statement (EOB/RA)

The EOB is the health carrier's way of finalizing a claim. The EOB is a detailed accounting of how the claim was processed and it should provide both balance and closure. Every line and every charge should be accounted for leaving you with a clear picture of how every dime of the bill claim was handled.

SAMPLE EOB

Patient Name: Test, Patient
Patient ID: 0000000000
Claim Number: QXXXXXXX
Processed Date: 1/27/16

Provider NPI: XXXXXXXXXX
Check Number:
EFT Number: 010121000
Check Amount: $104.00
Check issued date: 1/31/16

Claim Summary

Date of Service	Place of Service	Service code	Qty	Submitted charges	Allowed amount	Not payable	Plan Deductible	Patient Co-pay/Coinsurance	Remark Code(s)	Pt Responsibility	Plan Paid
01/01/2016	11	99213	1	$250.00	$155.00	$95.00	$50.00	$21.00	1,2	$71.00	$84.00
01/01/2016	11	81000	1	$25.00	$25.00			$5.00		$5.00	$20.00
Totals				**$275.00**	**$180.00**	**$95.00**	**$50.00**	**$26.00**		**$76.00**	**$104.00**

Remark Code (s) Detail:

1 - Participating provider charge is limited to the allowed amount- the patient is not responsible for this amount.

2. Changes applied to plan deductible - your calendar deductible has been met in full.

**** You have the right to request a reconsideration of this claim. You must file your request within 60 calendar days from the date on this Explanation of Benefit statement. You must include the reason for the request and all supporting documents, including any clinical data that fully supports your appeal. Mail all pertinent information to ABC Ins. Company, P.O Box 1000.

What each section means:

Date of Service - Date that the patient was seen by the provider of service.

Place of Service - Place where service was rendered; i.e., office, hospital, home, etc.

Service Code - The appropriate CPT-4/HCPCS codes that were billed to describe the services that were performed.

Qty. - The number of services/items that were performed or provided to the patient.

Submitted Charges - The total charge that was billed by the provider of service for that CPT-4/HCPCS code.

Allowed Amount - The total charges that the health carrier allowed for that CPT-4/HCPCS code.

Not Payable - Any amount deemed not payable by the health carrier. This includes amounts that exceed the allowed amount and any not covered charges.

Plan Deductible - Total amount that was applied to the plan deductible.

Pt. Copay/Coinsurance - The amount of the claim that the carrier has deemed to be patient liability.

Remark Code(s) - Because an EOB/RA lacks the space to fully explain every aspect of claim handling, a remark code is used to point you to the correct detailed explanation on how a claim was processed.

Pt Responsibility - The total amount that the patient is required to pay for this claim. This includes any copay, coinsurance, deductible or not covered amounts.

Plan Paid - The amount that the health carrier paid on this claim.

Remark Code(s) Detailed Description - An EOB/RA may have a section, below the Claim Summary Section that provides a detailed description of what each remark code(s) may mean or it may provide only the code and you would have to visit www.wpc.com to get the description.

The Appeal Information - This is usually provided as a note in the reason code section or it can be provided in full detail on the back of the EOB/RA.

The most important areas of any EOB include:

- Do the totals all add up and was every service accounted for?
- Is any amount not covered/or over the allowed amount?
- Provider payment and what is the patient responsibility.
- If underpaid, the remark codes will provide a clue as to why and how to proceed.

Note: Just like every health carrier is different, every EOB issued by a health carrier will be different. These differences will range from a simple ½ page EOB with minimal information to an EOB that has several pages of detail.

Finally: This sample EOB was designed to provide a basic overview of the information normally contained on an EOB/RA. Every health carrier's EOB will be different, but I am sure you will find that most of them will provide the same information that is found on this sample.

Rest assured, once you understand how to read this EOB, all others, no matter how different or detailed, will be fairly easy to unravel.

EOB's are excellent sources of data on allowed amounts. I keep a cheat sheet of my most common codes with the allowed amounts by carrier. This helps me to have some idea what will be allowed so I know what to collect upfront. This will not be exact, as reimbursement will differ, but this will get you fairly close.

HOW TO FOLLOW UP ON A CLAIM

Because of the awesome advances in technology, we can now easily and quickly:

- Confirm that a claim is on file with the health carrier.
- Obtain claim status.
- Question or dispute the way a claim was processed.
- Have a claim routed back for correction.

Sort your follow-ups into separate stacks, by health carrier. For example, you would put all of your calls to United HealthCare together, this way you can check the status on as many different patients as you can during the same call.

In a dream world, a claim is billed and 30 to 45 days later the correct payment just rolls right in.

Unfortunately, the real world scenario looks more like 60 plus days later with you still trying to move a claim to payment. So keeping your eye on the status of all claims is critical. Here are a few different options for claim follow up:

- Automated system
- The health carrier website
- The Clearinghouse
- Availity

Review your expectations for each claim before you call, this way if payment is not as expected you know to push for correction or, at least, an acceptable explanation.

Automated System

You now have the option to check status by phone. After a series of prompts, you will be connected with the automated system where you can speak or use the telephone key pad to enter your patient's ID number, date of birth, date of service and total charge and the provider's NPI number to obtain status on the claim in question.

The automated system will provide details about a processed claim, including paid dates and check amounts. You can also learn if a claim has been denied or if the claim is not on file.

The automated system is a fairly fast and easy way to obtain the information needed to help you resolve some claim issues. If the claim is not on file, you will know to rebill it and if the claim has been processed, you can simply wait for payment to arrive.

However, the automated system is not very effective for claims that have been denied since it does not provide the reason for denial nor does it tell you what steps you need to take to correct the claim. You will have to reach a live person for that level of information.

Health Carrier's Website

Most health carriers have a website that allows providers, even non-participating, access to RA's or EOB's to check claim status, patient eligibility or to submit additional information for a pending claim.

The carrier normally requires some type of enrollment process that may take a few weeks to complete. After enrollment is completed, you will be notified by the carrier.

Access to your billed claims is as simple as remembering your password and user ID.

Clearinghouse

If you bill claims through a clearinghouse and you receive EFT payments and EOB's electronically, the clearinghouse provides real time notification when a claim has been paid and when an EOB is on file.

You can easily access this information for review and disposition, including secondary billing, adjustments or write offs, claim disputes and appeals and patient invoicing.

Availity

Availity is the system where you can find remittance advice and claim information for patients with commercial plans, including Blue Cross Blue Shield, Humana and Cigna.

You are required to enroll, but once enrollment is completed you will be able to check claim status on tons of patients with various plans.

This system does fall short for denied claims as you will still need to call the carrier to get clear information on the reason for denial.

Pick any method you prefer, including speaking to a live person, just don't leave money on the table by failing to follow up timely.

Don't be afraid to ask for a supervisor if the information provided does not sit well with you. Recently, I had a Customer Service Rep from a large, well known carrier, tell me that they cannot fix my claim, despite admitting (finally) that it was paid incorrectly, because we cashed the check. After speaking with the supervisor, I was finally able to get my claim resolved.

HOW TO COMPLETE A CMS 1500 FORM

By now, you should fully understand WHY the billing process is so important. Billing a CMS 1500 claim form is the **only** way for providers to get reimbursed from health insurance carriers for the services they provide.

Unfortunately, HOW to complete a CMS is not so easy to pin down.

Over the pages of this guide, we have repeated the words, "every health insurance carrier is different, so the processes and procedures will be different," over and over again. I don't think this statement applies more than when it pertains to creating a CMS 1500 form.

Most medical billing software is designed to make the overall, generic creation of a CMS 1500 form fairly easy. You input the data and it is transposed into the correct fields on the form. For a good portion of your daily billing, this approach will work. But this will not work for ***all*** health carriers in ***all*** situations, ***all*** of the time. The key is knowing that at some point, you have to try something else.

In this section, we have provided the field descriptions and whether some inputs in that field are required or optional, again, because the data that a health carrier expects to see will differ. This pertains to only the accepted version of the CMS 1500 form, version 2/12. All other versions are no longer accepted by health insurance carriers. Use this section to:

- Become familiar with the fields on a CMS 1500 form.

- Learn what each field means and what type of data should be inputted into that field.
- Understand that the requirements for paper vs electronic claims may be different.
- Use the tips as a guide.
- Realize that every carrier is particular about what they expect their claim to look like.
- Understand that creation WILL NOT always result in payment. Claims will be kicked if the way the claim was billed isn't right. You are expected to figure out how to get this claim to payment.
- Know that this industry is ever-changing. There is no way that you will ever know everything. There is no shame is contacting the health carrier for assistance.

The way a CMS could be filled out will vary greatly. Keep a cheat sheet of requirements by carrier. When in doubt, almost every carrier has a billing manual online that can guide you through the process.

HEALTH INSURANCE CLAIM FORM

APPROVED BY NATIONAL UNIFORM CLAIM COMMITTEE (NUCC) 02/12

PICA　　　　PICA

CARRIER

1. MEDICARE (Medicare#) MEDICAID (Medicaid#) TRICARE (ID#/DoD#) CHAMPVA (Member ID#) GROUP HEALTH PLAN (ID#) FECA BLK LUNG (ID#) OTHER (ID#)

1a. INSURED'S I.D. NUMBER (For Program in Item 1)

2. PATIENT'S NAME (Last Name, First Name, Middle Initial)

3. PATIENT'S BIRTH DATE MM DD YY SEX M F

4. INSURED'S NAME (Last Name, First Name, Middle Initial)

5. PATIENT'S ADDRESS (No., Street)

6. PATIENT RELATIONSHIP TO INSURED Self Spouse Child Other

7. INSURED'S ADDRESS (No., Street)

CITY STATE

8. RESERVED FOR NUCC USE

CITY STATE

ZIP CODE TELEPHONE (Include Area Code) ( )

ZIP CODE TELEPHONE (Include Area Code) ( )

9. OTHER INSURED'S NAME (Last Name, First Name, Middle Initial)

10. IS PATIENT'S CONDITION RELATED TO:

11. INSURED'S POLICY GROUP OR FECA NUMBER

a. OTHER INSURED'S POLICY OR GROUP NUMBER

a. EMPLOYMENT? (Current or Previous) YES NO

a. INSURED'S DATE OF BIRTH MM DD YY SEX M F

b. RESERVED FOR NUCC USE

b. AUTO ACCIDENT? YES NO PLACE (State)

b. OTHER CLAIM ID (Designated by NUCC)

c. RESERVED FOR NUCC USE

c. OTHER ACCIDENT? YES NO

c. INSURANCE PLAN NAME OR PROGRAM NAME

d. INSURANCE PLAN NAME OR PROGRAM NAME

10d. CLAIM CODES (Designated by NUCC)

d. IS THERE ANOTHER HEALTH BENEFIT PLAN? YES NO *If yes*, complete items 9, 9a, and 9d.

READ BACK OF FORM BEFORE COMPLETING & SIGNING THIS FORM.

12. PATIENT'S OR AUTHORIZED PERSON'S SIGNATURE I authorize the release of any medical or other information necessary to process this claim. I also request payment of government benefits either to myself or to the party who accepts assignment below.

SIGNED ______ DATE ______

13. INSURED'S OR AUTHORIZED PERSON'S SIGNATURE I authorize payment of medical benefits to the undersigned physician or supplier for services described below.

SIGNED ______

PATIENT AND INSURED INFORMATION

14. DATE OF CURRENT ILLNESS, INJURY, or PREGNANCY (LMP) MM DD YY QUAL.

15. OTHER DATE QUAL. MM DD YY

16. DATES PATIENT UNABLE TO WORK IN CURRENT OCCUPATION FROM MM DD YY TO MM DD YY

17. NAME OF REFERRING PROVIDER OR OTHER SOURCE 17a. 17b. NPI

18. HOSPITALIZATION DATES RELATED TO CURRENT SERVICES FROM MM DD YY TO MM DD YY

19. ADDITIONAL CLAIM INFORMATION (Designated by NUCC)

20. OUTSIDE LAB? YES NO $ CHARGES

21. DIAGNOSIS OR NATURE OF ILLNESS OR INJURY Relate A-L to service line below (24E) ICD Ind.

A. B. C. D.
E. F. G. H.
I. J. K. L.

22. RESUBMISSION CODE ORIGINAL REF. NO.

23. PRIOR AUTHORIZATION NUMBER

24. A. DATE(S) OF SERVICE From MM DD YY To MM DD YY	B. PLACE OF SERVICE	C. EMG	D. PROCEDURES, SERVICES, OR SUPPLIES (Explain Unusual Circumstances) CPT/HCPCS MODIFIER	E. DIAGNOSIS POINTER	F. $ CHARGES	G. DAYS OR UNITS	H. EPSDT Family Plan	I. ID. QUAL.	J. RENDERING PROVIDER ID. #
1								NPI	
2								NPI	
3								NPI	
4								NPI	
5								NPI	
6								NPI	

PHYSICIAN OR SUPPLIER INFORMATION

25. FEDERAL TAX I.D. NUMBER SSN EIN

26. PATIENT'S ACCOUNT NO.

27. ACCEPT ASSIGNMENT? (For govt. claims, see back) YES NO

28. TOTAL CHARGE $

29. AMOUNT PAID $

30. Rsvd for NUCC Use

31. SIGNATURE OF PHYSICIAN OR SUPPLIER INCLUDING DEGREES OR CREDENTIALS (I certify that the statements on the reverse apply to this bill and are made a part thereof.)

SIGNED DATE

32. SERVICE FACILITY LOCATION INFORMATION a. b.

33. BILLING PROVIDER INFO & PH # ( ) a. b.

NUCC Instruction Manual available at: www.nucc.org　　*PLEASE PRINT OR TYPE*　　APPROVED OMB-0938-1197 FORM 1500 (02-12)

CMS 1500 form was retrieved from www.cms.gov.

Use the above picture of a CMS 1500 form for reference on how to complete numbers 1 – 33B

FIELD NUMBER	WHAT INFO SHOULD GO IN THAT FIELD	REQUIRED OR OPTIONAL
1	Plan type: Medicare/Medicaid/Tricare/ChampVA/ Group Plan/ Black Lung/Other	Optional or Required
1A	Insured ID Number	REQUIRED
2	Patient's Last Name, First Name	REQUIRED
3	Patient's Date of Birth	REQUIRED
4	Insured's Last Name, First Name	REQUIRED
5	Patient's address, City, State, Zip, Phone	REQUIRED
6	Patients Relationship to Insured: Self, Spouse, Child, Other	REQUIRED
7	Insured's Address, City, State, Zip, Phone	REQUIRED
8	Reserved- DO NOT USE	-
9	Other Insured Last Name, First Name- COB	Optional or Required
9A	Other Insured Policy or Group Number- COB	Optional or Required
9B	RESERVED - DO NOT USE	-
9C	RESERVED - DO NOT USE	-
9D	Other Insurance Carrier Name	Optional or Required
10A-C	Condition, Accident or Work Related	Required if applicable
11	Insured's Group Number	REQUIRED
11A	Insured's Date of Birth	REQUIRED
11B	RESERVED - DO NOT USE	-
11C	Insurance Carrier Name	Optional or Required
12	Authorization to Release Information	REQUIRED
13	Assignment of Benefits Who should get paid for this visit?	Depends on if visit was paid in full/part
14	Date of Current Illness	Optional or Required

15	Other Dates of Illnesses (other conditions)	Optional or Required
16	Date/s Patient was unable to work	Optional or Required for work comp claims
17	Name of Referring Provider	Optional or Required
17A	Referring Provider State License Number	Optional or Required
17B	Referring Provider NPI Number	Optional or Required
18	Hospital Admission/Discharge Dates	Optional or Required
19	This field is to add info or notes about the claim	Optional or Required
20	Outside Lab – Yes or No	Optional or Required
21A-L	ICD-10 Codes – 12 different illness/diagnosis/injury codes can be added. One on each letter A-L	REQUIRED
22	Resubmission code – if this is a rebilling of same claim	Optional or Required
23	Prior Authorization (PA) Number	Required if PA was Obtained
24A	Date of Service	REQUIRED
24B	Place of Service	REQUIRED
24C	Emergency Indicator	Optional or Required
24D	CPT/HCPCS/MODIFIER Codes	REQURIED
24E	DIAG POINTER – Points to A-L in Field 21	REQUIRED
24F	Billed Charge	REQUIRED
24G	Total number of services	REQUIRED
24H	EPSDT	If Applicable
24I	ID Qualifier – Billing Emergency Services	If Applicable
24J	Rendering Provider NPI Number	If Applicable
25	Provider's Federal Tax ID Number	REQUIRED
26	Patient Account Number	Optional or Required
27	Accept Assignment	If Applicable

28	Total Charge	REQUIRED
29	Amount Paid	If Applicable
30	RESERVED - DO NOT USE	-
31	Signature of Provider of Service (or representative) sign in Black Ink	REQUIRED
32	Place of Service Address, City, State, Zip - where services were preformed	Optional or Required
32A	Place of Service NPI number	Optional or Required
32B	Place of Service Provider Number – could be Medicaid/Taxonomy number	Optional or Required
33	Billing Provider Address, City, State, Zip	REQUIRED
33A	Billing Provider NPI Number	REQUIRED
33B	Billing Provider Number – could be Medicaid/Taxonomy number	Optional or Required

This interpretation of how to complete a CMS 1500 form is merely a guide. Please refer to the health carrier's website if you have questions on how to complete your specific CMS 1500 form.

Since every carrier is different, what is required or optional information could vary. What one carrier uses as required, another carrier may deem optional. Health carriers are very particular about how this form is completed but over the years, I have developed my own "standard" way to bill paper and electronic claims:

PAPER CLAIMS

- The ink must be dark enough to be visible after scanning. Refresh all old printer cartridges.
- No hand written fields (other than a signature in box 31)
- Keep within the fields.
- No blue, red or any other colored ink.
- All data must fit squarely in each field.
- Be careful with your fonts. Times New Roman seems to be the preferred font.
- Use no mixed fonts. Stick with one, i.e., italicized, bold, small text, large text, caps, etc., for the full form
- No special characters, i.e., dashes, hyphens, number signs etc.
- Mail no more than 3-4 in one envelope.
- No staples
- ICD indicator (field 21) must be 9 for ICD-9 and 0 for ICD-10

ELECTRONIC

- The patient name must match the patient name on the ID card exactly. For example, Elizabeth on the ID card but claim is billed as Beth.
- The patient and insured dates of birth, sex, and ID numbers must be the same information that is on file with the health carrier.
- The NPI must match the provider.
- Referring/ordering provider is mandatory for certain services.
- The zip codes must be correct (this is a new reason for rejection).

HOW TO ISSUE AN ABN FORM

An Advanced Beneficiary Notice (ABN) is a form that is required by the Centers for Medicare & Medicaid Services (CMS) as a way to notify Medicare beneficiaries that an item or service that is usually covered, may not be paid for by Medicare for some reason.

This way the Medicare beneficiary can make an informed decision about whether or not they want to proceed with the treatment, service or supply.

The ABN form CMS-R-131 is used for patients with original or traditional Medicare ONLY. Go to www.cms.gov for a copy of the ABN form. Patients with managed care plans must be issued a denial notice which fully explains the reason for non-coverage and any appeal rights.

An ABN is required if:

- You believe Medicare may not pay for an item or service.
- Medicare usually covers the item or service but you expect them to deny payment because it is not medically necessary or it exceeds guidelines for coverage.

A Medicare Beneficiary ***cannot*** be held financially responsible if a provider fails to get an ABN form signed, ***in advance***, and Medicare does not pay.

A Medicare beneficiary must sign the form even if they verbally agree to provide payment upfront and they claim that they fully understand that payment may not be forthcoming.

If an ABN is required, while the patient is still in the office, advise them that the item or service may not be covered and the reason. Have them sign a Medicare approved ABN form. They will need to choose either option 1 or 2:

- Option One: I understand that Medicare may not pay for this item or service for the stated reason - **But bill Medicare anyway.**
- Option Two – I understand that Medicare may not pay for this item or service for the stated reason - **Do not bill Medicare.**

Once it is signed, you can request payment in full upfront.

Based on the selected option the claim may be billed to Medicare. If Medicare pays all or part of the claim, the provider is required to issue a refund to the Medicare beneficiary in a timely manner. Per Medicare, a refund is considered timely when they are made within 30 days after you receive the Remittance Advice from Medicare.

If the **beneficiary refuses to choose an option or sign the ABN**, you can note that the patient refused to sign the form but Medicare suggests that you should consider not furnishing the item or service unless the patient's health or safety is in jeopardy.

Note: An ABN is not needed for services/items that are listed as not covered by Medicare.

ABN Modifiers

A modifier is used as a footnote to a claim and is designed to provide the claim processor with a bit more information about the claim. These modifiers can be used in a ABN situation:

Modifier GA - ***Waiver of Liability Statement Issued as Required by Payer Policy, Individual Case.***

- Report when you issue a mandatory ABN for a service as required and it is on file. You do not need to submit a copy of the ABN, but you must have it available on request.

Modifier GX - ***Notice of Liability Issued, Voluntary Under Payer Policy.***

- Report when you issue a voluntary ABN for a service Medicare never covers because it is statutorily excluded or is not a Medicare benefit. You may use this modifier in combination with modifier GY.

Modifier GY - ***Item or Service Statutorily Excluded Does Not Meet the Definition of Any Medicare Benefit.***

- Report that Medicare statutorily excludes the item or service or the item or service does not meet the definition of any Medicare benefit. You may use this modifier in combination with modifier GX.

Modifier GZ - ***Item or Service Expected to Be Denied as Not Reasonable and Necessary*** .

- Report when you expect Medicare to deny payment of the item or service due to a lack of medical necessity and no ABN was issued.

HOW TO BILL SECONDARY AND TERTIARY CLAIMS

For patients with more than one health plan, you may need to bill **all** carriers, one after the other, in order to be reimbursed the full amount that is due.

Step One

Make sure you have the complete coverage and billing information on all carriers. The patient is responsible for providing full disclosure on all health carriers. For some reason, a patient may feel they have the option to pick and choose the information they provide.

Step Two

Determine which health carrier is primary. This is not always cut and dry. Refer to Chapter Eight, "How To Determine Who to Bill First," for help figuring this out.

Step Three

Once you determine who to bill first, create the CMS 1500 claim as you normally would with the primary insurance information in the appropriate fields.

For Example

John J. is covered under two health plans, a Medicare plan that is primary and a Medicaid that is secondary. The primary claim is created first. This claim will reflect the member ID and group numbers as well as the billing address of the Medicare plan. The claim is then billed to the primary carrier.

Step Four

Wait for the claim to be processed by the primary carrier. You will need the EOB from the primary to bill secondary.

Step Five

The EOB is received, reviewed and all required adjustments are cleared off the account. If a balance still remains, you are ready to bill the secondary carrier.

You are required to adjust off all amounts that exceed the contracted rates or the Medicare or Medicaid allowed amounts. These amounts will not be considered by a secondary plan. You can bill for any over allowed amounts if you are nonparticipating.

Example #1:

Dr. Eden is a **participating provider** who treats a patient with two health plans. The patient incurs $1000.00 in charges. Primary EOB looks like this:

$1000.00 claim

$500.00 denied as over allowed

$500.00 allowed amount

$500.00 paid at 100%

$500.00 paid to provider

In this scenario, the secondary plan will not be billed because the claim is paid in full, with $500.00 going to write off.

Example #2:

Dr. Eden is a **non-participating provider** who treats a patient with two health plans. The patient incurs $1000.00 in charges. Primary EOB looks like this:

$1000.00 claim

$500.00 denied as over allowed

$500.00 allowed amount

$500.00 paid at 100%

$500.00 paid to provider

In this scenario, because the provider is out of network, he is not required to write off the $500.00 that exceeded the allowed amount. The secondary plan will be billed with the EOB showing a payment of $500.00 and we expect the remaining $500.00 balance to be paid by the secondary plan.

If the primary carrier's payment is not as expected, you should dispute the payment before you bill the secondary carrier.

Step Six

A second CMS 1500 claim is created, almost identical to the one that was created for the primary claim, except that the secondary insurance information is entered and field 29 will include any payments that were made by the primary carrier.

The claim is printed and mailed to the secondary health carrier with a copy of the primary EOB. The secondary carrier will use the EOB to determine what, if any, they will pay on that claim.

Note: If you have the ability to upload a copy of the EOB and submit it electronically it is the preferred method. But most carriers still require a copy of the EOB and claim by mail.

Step Seven

The secondary EOB is received, hopefully, with the full payment that was expected. If it is not paid as expected and a balance remains, the EOB will be reviewed to determine if:

- The claim requires correction or supporting documents before it is rebilled.
- A balance is deemed to be due from the patient. The patient would then be invoiced and the file flagged if the account is outstanding.
- The carrier information on file is incorrect. The patient would then be contacted to update the insurance information.
- The balance is a write off.

- A tertiary carrier should be billed using the same process.

Timely filing starts from the date the primary claim was processed . It does not start from the day you decide to bill the secondary.

HOW TO DETERMINE WHO TO BILL FIRST

Determining the primary insurance carrier is not always clear and the rules may not always be cut and dry. The following represents just some of the more common scenarios for patients with more than one health carrier.

Use this as a guide only, as the COB rules may differ by health carrier, by court mandate and even by state. When in doubt, refer to the carrier for clarification.

Married/Living Together (Intact Family)

Both parents work Both have group health plans where they insure themselves, spouse and any kids.	• Each parent would be primary under their own plan. • For the children the **Birthday Rule** applies - the parent with the earlier birthday is prime. Example: Mom's birthday is April and Dad's is September - so mom is primary. • If they have the same birthday then the policy that has been in effect the longest is primary.
One person has Medicare and also is covered under a spouse who has a group plan with more than 20 employees.	• The group plan would be primary and Medicare is secondary.
One has Medicare and is also covered under a spouse who has a group plan with less than 20 employees.	• Medicare is primary and the group plan is secondary.
One person has Tri-care and the other person has a group health plan.	• The group plan would be primary. • Tricare is **always** secondary to any plan.
A working employee and retired employee both with group plans.	• The working plan is primary.
One person has Medicaid and the other person has a group health plan.	• The group plan would be primary. • Medicaid is always secondary to any plan.

Divorced Couples

Parents are divorced and a decree has addressed this issue.	• Whoever the divorce decree has mandated as primary will pay first.
Child resides with one parent.	• The parent that has custody is primary. Noncustodial parent is secondary.
Parents have shared custody so child resides in two homes.	• The birthday rule would apply.
Step children	• Would go according to divorce decree or custodial. The stepparent is always last.

Single Person with More Than One Health Plan

Two jobs and two group plans	• The plan that has been in affect longer is primary.
Group plan and Medicaid	• Group plan is always primary.
Group and Tricare	• Group plan is always primary.
Group and individual plan	• Group plan is primary.

CHAPTER EIGHT TEST

Directions: Using what you have learned in Chapter Eight, answer the following questions.

1. What are the two questions that the PCP must answer before a referral is granted?

2. Why will health insurance carriers issue a pre-approval letter that includes a disclaimer that the approval is not a guarantee of payment?

3. How many levels of appeal does Medicare offer?

4. Is the appeal process the same for all Medicaid plans?

5. Why should you get a reference number when calling a health carrier's Customer Service Department?.

6. A patient has been coming to the office for years, do you need to keep verifying benefits?

7. You called to verify benefits but do you also need to read the Benefit Booklet?

8. Why would you need to go to www.wpc- edi.com?

9. What version of the CMS 1500 form is the only acceptable version?

10. If the patients refused to sign an ABN what should you do?

9 INDUSTRY INFORMATION

Chapter Overview – The health insurance industry has its own unique terminology, acronyms, definitions and general information. In this chapter, you will have access to all of this need-to-know information.

This Chapter Includes:

Common Industry Terms and Definitions

Acronyms

COMMON INDUSTRY TERMS & INFORMATION

Adjudication

All of the various processes that a claim goes through, once it reaches the health carrier, that will result in the final disposition of that claim.

Allowed amount, allowable amount or allowable charge

The maximum amount that the plan will pay for a service or procedure.

Appeal

Request that a health carrier take a second look at the way they handled a claim for the purpose of having it reprocessed.

Assignment

Permission to pay all claim payments directly to the provider of service.

Authorization

Health carrier has given permission, before it is rendered, for a patient to have a requested service, treatment or supply.

Balance billing

Billing a patient for any amount that remains on account after the health carrier has paid its portion.

Beneficiary

The term that a person covered under Medicare plan is called.

CHAMPUS

Civilian Health and Medical Program of the Uniformed Service is the plan that provides coverage to our military and their families.

Claim

The bill that is submitted to the health carrier that details all aspects of a patients encounter with a medical provider.

COBRA

Consolidated Omnibus Budget Reconciliation Act

Coinsurance

The portion that a patient is required to pay out of pocket.

Concurrent Review

Monitoring a patient, while they are still hospital-confined, as a way to ensure that they are in the most cost effective level of care.

Continuity of Care

The ability to continue the current care in spite of a coverage, plan or benefit change.

Coordination of Benefits

The process of determining how claims will be billed when a person has more than one health plan.

Copayment

The portion that a patient is required to pay out of pocket.

Credentialing

The process of verifying and accepting a health care provider before they are allowed to participate as an in network provider.

Deductible

The portion that members must first pay before the health plan will start to pay.

ERISA

Employment Retirement Income Security Act

Explanation of Benefits

A statement that is issued by a health insurance carrier that explains how a claim was processed.

Explanation of Medicare Benefits

A statement that is issued by Medicare that explains how a Medicare claim was processed.

Family Deductible

The combined maximum that a family is required to pay out of pocket before the health plan will start to pay.

Fee-For-Service

Charges billed by the provider on a per service basis.

Fee Schedule

A list that of allowed amounts by CPT-4/HCPCS code.

Group

All of the employees that are covered under the employer's health plan.

HCFA-1500 Claim

The claim form that is used to bill professional (non-hospital) services to insurance carriers.

HCPCS codes

Alphanumeric codes that are used to bill ambulance services, durable medical equipment and other non-physician type services.

HIPAA

Health Insurance Portability and Accountability Act

HMO

A plan that contracts with medical providers to provide restricted access care only to patients.

Home Plan

The Blue Cross and Blue Shield plan where the member is enrolled.

Host Plan

The Blue Cross and Blue Shield plan that services the out of area member.

ICD-9

The International Classification of Diseases, 9th edition - Clinical Modification manual.

Limiting Charge

115% of the Medicare allowed amount is all that a nonparticipating provider is allowed to charge a Medicare patient.

Managed Care

The process of controlling health care costs by controlling how heath care is delivered.

Mandated Benefits

A type of benefit, provision or coverage that must be offered by law.

Medicaid

Health insurance coverage available to persons who become eligible because they are disabled or have low-income.

Medicare

Health insurance coverage available to persons 65 or older, disabled or with end stage renal disease.

Medigap

An additional health plan that is available to Medicare beneficiaries with Medicare 80/20 plans as a way to offset out of pocket costs.

Member

Person that is enrolled in a health insurance plan.

Modifier

A code that is added to the claim when billing as way to further describe or explain an encounter.

Network

A group of medical providers, of all specialties, that are under contract with a health insurance carrier for the purpose of providing care to plan members at reduced rates.

Nonparticipating Providers

A provider that refuses to contract with any health insurance carrier.

Open Enrollment

The period, normally once per year, where a plan member can switch from one plan to another, if offered.

Out-of-Network services

Services performed by a provider who refuses to contract with a health insurance carrier.

Participating Provider

Providers that are under contract with a health insurance carrier.

Point of Service

A plan where the patient has the freedom to choose, at the time they need care, how they wish to have it delivered.

PPO

A plan that is designed to encourage plan members to use under-contract providers resulting in lower out of pocket and higher reimbursement.

Preapproval

Health carrier has given permission for a patient to have a requested service, treatment or supply.

Preauthorization

Health carrier has given permission for a patient to have a requested service, treatment or supply.

Precertification

Health carrier has given permission for a patient to have a hospital related service.

Primary Care Physician (PCP)

A medical provider that is tasked with overseeing all aspects of a patient's care.

Procedure Code

Numeric or alphanumeric billing codes that describe all medical services.

Provider

Person or facility where one can receive medical care.

Referral

Permission for a member to obtain specialty or out of network care.

Reimbursement

Payment for medical services that were rendered to a plan member.

Retrospective Review

A review of all services after they have been rendered.

Self-Funded Plan

A group plan where the employer is responsible for funding all claims that are incurred by the employees/dependents

Subrogation

Refund of all money that was paid by a health carrier for claims incurred due to a negligent third party.

Third-Party Administrator

A company responsible for all claim related tasks.

Traditional Coverage

A medical plan that designed to include a preset level of cost sharing between health insurance carrier and plan member.

Unbundling

Breaking down a service, treatment or supply into numerous different charges when it should have been included, all together, as one charge.

Usual, Customary and Reasonable Charge

Refers to the way that a health insurance carrier will re-price a claim to the most average or usual charge for a particular service, treatment or supply.

Utilization Review

Monitoring or overseeing all aspects of a patient's care as a way to control costs.

ACRONYMS

Acronym	Definition
AA	Allowed Amount
ABN	Advance Beneficiary Notice
AR	Accounts Receivable
ASF	Ambulatory Surgical Facilities
BAA	Business Associate Agreement
BCBS	Blue Cross Blue Shield
CMN	Certificate of Medical Necessity
CMS	Centers for Medicare and Medicaid Services
COB	Coordination of benefits
COBRA	Consolidated Omnibus Budget Reconciliation Act
CPT	Current Procedural Terminology
DME	Durable Medical Equipment
DMEPOS	Durable Medical Equipment, Prosthetics, Orthotics and Supplies
DOL	Date of Loss

DOS	Date of Service
DRG	Diagnosis Related Group
EDI	Electronic Data Interchange
EFI	Electronic Funds Transfer data interchange
EOB	Explanation of Benefits
EOMB	Explanation of Medicare Benefits
EPO	Exclusive Provider Organization
ERISA	Employer Retirement Income Security Act
ESRD	End Stage Renal Disease
FFS	Fee for Service
GHP	Group Health Plan
HCPCS	Healthcare Common Procedure Coding System
HHA	Home Health Agency
HHS	U.S. Department of Health and Human Services
HIC	Health Insurance Claim
HIPAA	Health Insurance Portability and Accountability Act of 1996
HMO	Health Maintenance Organization
ICD-9	International Classification of Disease, Ninth edition
ICD-10	International Classification of Disease, Tenth edition
ID	Identification
LCD	Local coverage determination

LOA	Letter of Agreement
MA	Medicare Advantage
MCP	Managed Care Plan
MDC	Medicare
MN	Medical Necessity
NCD	National Coverage Determination
NPI	National Provider Identifier
OON	Out of Network
OOP	Out of Pocket
OPPS	Outpatient Prospective Payment System
P&O	Prosthetic and Orthotics
PA	Pre-Approval/Preauthorization
Part A	Hospital Insurance Provided by Medicare
Part B	Medical Insurance Provided by Medicare
Part D	Prescription Drug Insurance Provided by Medicare
PCP	Primary Care Physician
PD	Pre Determination
PFFS	Private Fee-For-Service plan
PHI	Protected Health Information
PMPM	Per Member Per Month

POS	Place of Service
POS	Point of Service
PPO	Preferred Provider Organization
QE	Qualifying Event
RA	Remittance Advice
RAP	Request for Anticipated Payment
RHC	Rural Health Clinic
RM	Revenue Management

CHAPTER NINE TEST

Directions: Using what you have learned in Chapter Nine, match the correct term to the appropriate definition.

	Credentialing	A	National Provider Identification Number.
	Assignment	B	All of the various processes that a claim goes through once it reaches the health carrier that will result in the final disposition of that claim.
	Limiting Charge	C	Breaking down a service, treatment, or supply into numerous different charges when it should have included, all together, as one charge.
	Open Enrollment	D	The process of verifying and accepting a healthcare provider before they being allowed to participate as an in network provider.
	Mandated Benefits	E	Medicare coverage for professional services.
	Unbundling	F	A type of benefit, provision or coverage that must be offered by law.
	NPI	G	115% of the Medicare allowed amount is all that non-participating provider is allowed to charge a Medicare patient.
	Adjudication	H	The period, normally once per year, where a plan member can switch from one plan to another, if offered.
	Part B	I	Advance Beneficiary Notice
	ABN	J	Permission to pay all claim payments directly to the provider of service.

SUMMARY

SUMMARY

We have reached the end of the 1500pays: A Health Insurance Guide, so let's go over this one last time - from initial contact to reconciliation.

Please note: "Observations" are simply the things most important about each phase of the process. I have included a real world example. So let's go through this step by step.

INSURANCE VERIFICATION FORM - PRIMARY

Patient Information

Today's Date: 06/16/16 **Patient Name:** Test, Patient **M/F:** M **DOB:** 09/09/99

Insured Name: Same as Above (SAA) **Insured DOB:** SAA ***Relationship to Patient*:** SAA

Member ID Number: P100PXXXXXXXXXX-01 **Group Number:** 123456XX

Plan Information

Plan Type: __HMO _X_ PPO __ EPO___ POS ___ Medicare ___ Medicaid ___Tricare __ Other

Insurance Carrier Name: The Ins Company **Phone:** (000) 000- 0000 **Effective Date:** 01/01/16

Address: *PO BOX 1234* ***City:*** XXXXX ***State:*** XYX **Zip:** 00000-0000

Benefits

	IN NETWORK	AMOUNT MET	OUT OF NET	AMOUNT MET
Deductible	0		$ 500.00	$150.00
Coinsurance	80/20		60/40	
OOP/Stop Loss	$1000.00 Individual $3000.00 family	0	$3000.00 individual $6000.00 Family	0
Plan Limits				
Lifetime Max	2 million		2 million	

General

Pre-Approval Required: Y or N *PA required if over $1000.00, all hospital and all MRI/CT scans.*
Referral Required: Y or (N) **UR phone:** (000) XXX-XXXX **Fax:** (000) XXX-XXX2
Provider in Network: (Y) or N **EDI Submitter#:** AZYYYY **Timely:** 180 days **CRS Name:** J Smith
Reference number: 216516416 **Form completed by:** M.E
Expectations: Pt to pay 20% of all orders upfront check history for allowed amts.
Comments: Patient has no secondary plan.

STEP 1: VERIFY BENEFITS ON ALL NEW PATIENTS AND ALL NEW PLANS.

Using the above Verification Form, we know that:

- The patient has a PPO plan no other coverage.
- No referral is required.
- No in network deductible and $500.00 out of net deductible.
- Pt to pay 20% upfront (in net) and 40% upfront (out of net).
- Carrier to pay 80% (in net) and 60% (out of net).
- Provider is in network.
- Pre-approval required for all claim amounts over $1000.00.
- Payment based on contracted rates.
- Balance over allowed is write off.

Expectations: Carrier to pay 80% of allowed/Patient to pay 20% of allowed. Claim not expected to go over $1000.00

PATIENT FILE

Pt Name: Test, Patient

DOB: 9/1/55

DATE: 6/1/2016

5/31/16: Pt called for appointment - scheduled for 6/1/16 at 2pm. Pt has PPO plan with the INS Company.

6/1/16 - T/c to The Insurance Company – patient eligible for coverage- see Ins Verification Form for plan information.

Vitals

B/P: 120/72

Height: 6.1

Weight: 189lb

Pt History and Physical

The patient a 60 year old male who is in office today complaining about chest pain and frequent heartburn, trouble swallowing and sour taste in mouth. Patient has a PPO plan. No other coverage.

Pt is in no distress today, he is a recreational weight lifter and is concerned about intermittent pain in his middle chest and throat area that that averages a 5-6 on the pain scale. Heartburn and pain after meals, especially spicy meals. Pt takes no medication.

Chest X-ray and EKG all normal.

Diagnosis: Chest pain due to heartburn/acid reflux. Possible Hiatal Hernia. Patient to be referred for Endoscopy to confirm diagnosis of Hiatal Hernia. Medication and return in 2 weeks for follow up.

Coding

ICD-10	HCPCS 1
Chest pain: R07.9	Exam 99203 $200.00
Acid Reflux: K21.9	Chest X- ray 71020 two view $75.00
Heartburn: R12	EKG 93000 complete $675.00

Patient released – prescriptions, referral for Endoscopy and follow up appointment in two weeks.

STEP 2: MAKE SURE THE PATIENT FILE SUPPORTS YOUR BILLED CLAIM.

Using the above notes in the patient's file, we know that:

- All billing codes fit the diagnosis and the services that were rendered.
- Patient complaints are clearly documented in the patient file.
- Patient treatment, is clearly documented in the patient file
- Possible Hiatal Hernia was not coded because you should code only what you know to be true. The patient has chest pain, acid reflux and heartburn- the hernia is yet to be confirmed.

Expectations: All codes should be payable as they are medically necessary and appropriate based on the patients complaints and the diagnosis.

HEALTH INSURANCE CLAIM FORM

APPROVED BY NATIONAL UNIFORM CLAIM COMMITTEE (NUCC) 02/12

THE INSURANCE COMPANY
ATTENTION: CLAIM DEPARTMENT
PO BOX 1234
XXXX XX 00000-0000

PICA — CARRIER — PICA

1. MEDICARE (Medicare#) | MEDICAID (Medicaid#) | TRICARE (ID#/DoD#) | CHAMPVA (Member ID#) | GROUP HEALTH PLAN (ID#) [X] | FECA BLK LUNG (ID#) | OTHER (ID#)

1a. INSURED'S I.D. NUMBER (For Program in Item 1): P100PXXXXXXXXXX-01

2. PATIENT'S NAME (Last Name, First Name, Middle Initial): TEST, PATIENT

3. PATIENT'S BIRTH DATE MM DD YY: 09 09 1999 SEX M [X] F [ ]

4. INSURED'S NAME (Last Name, First Name, Middle Initial): TEST, PATIENT

5. PATIENT'S ADDRESS (No., Street): 42 WEST YYYYY

6. PATIENT RELATIONSHIP TO INSURED: Self [X] Spouse [ ] Child [ ] Other [ ]

7. INSURED'S ADDRESS (No., Street): 42 WEST YYYYY

CITY: XXXXX STATE: XX

8. RESERVED FOR NUCC USE

CITY: XXXXX STATE: XX

ZIP CODE: XXXXX-XXXX TELEPHONE (Include Area Code): (111) 1111111

ZIP CODE: XXXXX-XXXX TELEPHONE (Include Area Code): (111) 1111111

9. OTHER INSURED'S NAME (Last Name, First Name, Middle Initial)

10. IS PATIENT'S CONDITION RELATED TO:

11. INSURED'S POLICY GROUP OR FECA NUMBER: 123456XX

a. OTHER INSURED'S POLICY OR GROUP NUMBER

a. EMPLOYMENT? (Current or Previous) [ ] YES [X] NO

a. INSURED'S DATE OF BIRTH MM DD YY: 09 09 1999 SEX M [X] F [ ]

b. RESERVED FOR NUCC USE

b. AUTO ACCIDENT? [ ] YES [X] NO PLACE (State)

b. OTHER CLAIM ID (Designated by NUCC)

c. RESERVED FOR NUCC USE

c. OTHER ACCIDENT? [ ] YES [X] NO

c. INSURANCE PLAN NAME OR PROGRAM NAME

d. INSURANCE PLAN NAME OR PROGRAM NAME

10d. CLAIM CODES (Designated by NUCC)

d. IS THERE ANOTHER HEALTH BENEFIT PLAN? [ ] YES [X] NO *If yes, complete items 9, 9a, and 9d.*

READ BACK OF FORM BEFORE COMPLETING & SIGNING THIS FORM.

12. PATIENT'S OR AUTHORIZED PERSON'S SIGNATURE I authorize the release of any medical or other information necessary to process this claim. I also request payment of government benefits either to myself or to the party who accepts assignment below.

SIGNED SIGNATURE ON FILE DATE 06 01 2016

13. INSURED'S OR AUTHORIZED PERSON'S SIGNATURE I authorize payment of medical benefits to the undersigned physician or supplier for services described below.

SIGNED SIGNATURE ON FILE

14. DATE OF CURRENT ILLNESS, INJURY, or PREGNANCY (LMP) MM DD YY: 06 01 2016 QUAL.

15. OTHER DATE QUAL. MM DD YY

16. DATES PATIENT UNABLE TO WORK IN CURRENT OCCUPATION FROM TO

17. NAME OF REFERRING PROVIDER OR OTHER SOURCE 17a. 17b. NPI

18. HOSPITALIZATION DATES RELATED TO CURRENT SERVICES FROM TO

19. ADDITIONAL CLAIM INFORMATION (Designated by NUCC)

20. OUTSIDE LAB? [ ] YES [X] NO $ CHARGES

21. DIAGNOSIS OR NATURE OF ILLNESS OR INJURY Relate A-L to service line below (24E) ICD Ind. 0

A. R07.9 B. K21.9 C. R12 D.
E. F. G. H.
I. J. K. L.

22. RESUBMISSION CODE ORIGINAL REF. NO.

23. PRIOR AUTHORIZATION NUMBER

	24. A. DATE(S) OF SERVICE From MM DD YY	To MM DD YY	B. PLACE OF SERVICE	C. EMG	D. PROCEDURES, SERVICES, OR SUPPLIES CPT/HCPCS	MODIFIER	E. DIAGNOSIS POINTER	F. $ CHARGES	G. DAYS OR UNITS	H. EPSDT Family Plan	I. ID. QUAL.	J. RENDERING PROVIDER ID. #
1	06 01 16	06 01 16	11		99203		ABC	200 00			NPI	0000000000
2	06 01 16	06 01 16	11		71020		ABC	75 00			NPI	0000000000
3	06 01 16	06 01 16	11		93000		ABC	675 00			NPI	0000000000
4											NPI	
5											NPI	
6											NPI	

25. FEDERAL TAX I.D. NUMBER: 333333333 SSN [ ] EIN [X]

26. PATIENT'S ACCOUNT NO.: ABCD123

27. ACCEPT ASSIGNMENT? (For govt. claims, see back) [X] YES [ ] NO

28. TOTAL CHARGE: $ 950 00

29. AMOUNT PAID: $ 190 00

30. Rsvd for NUCC Use

31. SIGNATURE OF PHYSICIAN OR SUPPLIER INCLUDING DEGREES OR CREDENTIALS (I certify that the statements on the reverse apply to this bill and are made a part thereof.)

THE DOCTOR SIGNED DATE 06012016

32. SERVICE FACILITY LOCATION INFORMATION: THE DOCTOR 12 WEST YYYYY STREET XXXXX XX 000000000 a. b.

33. BILLING PROVIDER INFO & PH # ( ): THE DOCTOR 12 WEST YYYYY STREET XXXXX XX 000000000 a. 3213213219 b.

NUCC Instruction Manual available at: www.nucc.org PLEASE PRINT OR TYPE APPROVED OMB-0938-1197 FORM 1500 (02-12)

PATIENT AND INSURED INFORMATION — PHYSICIAN OR SUPPLIER INFORMATION

STEP 3: CREATE A CMS 1500 FORM.

Using the verification form and the Pt. file, the CMS 1500 is created and:

- All required fields were completed.
- The ICD-10 and CPT-4 codes are correct as supported in the patient record.
- Signature on file authorizes payment to the doctor.

Expectations: Clean claim was created that should result in correct payment at first billing.

THE INSURANCE COMPANY

1234 West XXXX

XXXXX, XX XXXXX-XXX

Provider NPI: 3213213219
Check Number: M1268
EFT Number:
Check Amount: $716.00
Check issued date: 7/1/2016

Patient name: Test, Patient
Patient ID: 31400032100001
Claim Number: 2121412
Processed Date: 07/01/2016

EOB- Explanation of Benefit

Date of Service	Place of Service	Service code	Units	Submitted charges	Allowed amount	Not payable	Reason Remark code	Deductible	Pt Responsibility	Payment Amount
06/01/16	11	99203	1	$200.00	$175.00	$25.00	1		$35.00	$140.00
06/01/16	11	71020	1	$75.00	$45.00	30.00	1		$9.00	$36.00
06/01/16	11	93000	1	$675.00	$675.00				$135.00	$540.00
Totals				**$950.00**	**$895.00**	**$55.00**			**$179.00**	**$716.00**

Remarks

1 - Participating provider charge is limited to the allowed amount- the patient is not responsible for the difference.

Detach and retain this stub for your records

The Ins. Company

No. 00000212

Pay to the order Of: The Doctor, MD

$716.00

STEP 4: REVIEW THE EOB.

Using the above EOB, we know that:

- Claim paid at correct plan percentage of 80%
- All codes were paid- no denied services
- $55.00 over allowed amount - to write off.
- Allowed amounts for these codes are added to the cheat sheet for future reference.
- Pt due a refund.

Expectation: Claim paid as expected, all lines accounted for.

<u>**STEP 5: RECONCILE THE ACCOUNT.**</u>

Billed: $950.00
Allowed: $895.00
Pt. paid: $190.00
Carrier paid: $716.00
Total paid: $906.00

Expectations: Patient due a refund of $11.00. Patient responsibility was $179.00 they paid $190.00.

CASE STUDY

Medical billers are like detectives and their claims can often be like cases. Most claims are simple with no real twists or turns. Others can be like a puzzle where you must revisit the evidence in order to find the clue that cracks the case wide open. Do you have what it takes to resolve a claim?

This Section Includes:

Case Study 1

Directions: Read the scenario below and answer any questions that follow. State your reasoning and any evidence to back up you answer.

THE CASE OF THE PREEXISTING CONDITION

Ashton quit his job at Soto School District on Friday, March 28, 2014 and began working for Sierra Social Services Agency effective March 31, 2014.

When he was hired at Sierra, he was aware that he would have to wait 90 days in order to begin receiving medical benefits. Ashton has high blood pressure that is controlled by daily medication but he opted not to enroll in Soto's COBRA insurance program because of the high cost. He was confident that he had enough refills to carry him through the 90 day waiting period.

The waiting period was uneventful. No medical services were needed other than medication refills and on July 1, 2014 Ashton's health coverage became effective.

Ashton visited his doctor on July 15, 2014 in order to get refills for his high blood pressure medication. At that time, his doctor requested labs to monitor his A1C levels. Ashton paid his copay before exiting the doctor's office and then went down the hall to give blood.

Since his doctor was in network he assumed that claim would be processed at the in network benefit level leaving him with no further financial liability so he was shocked, when in September, he received a bill for $722.00 for office/lab fees that were incurred on July 15, 2014. His claim had been denied because his high blood pressure was deemed to be a pre-existing condition. He was given 20 days to appeal the denial.

Ashton immediately calls his friend Riley, who works in the insurance business and she informs him that the Affordable Care Act banned Pre Existing exclusions and that health insurers were no longer able to deny claims based on this. Riley suggests that he file an appeal immediately. After hanging up, Ashton does some research of his own online and his findings seem to heavily support what his friend Riley has said. So Ashton prints his documents and begins drafting his appeal.

Ashton submits his appeal well within the allotted time and waits for follow up. Fifteen days later he receives a letter from his insurance company which states that his appeal is denied due to the described reasons.

How was his insurance company able to justify his denial?

See the answer on page 372

Case Study 2

Directions: Examine the information provided below and answer the questions that follow. Use what you have learned about plan types to help you arrive at your answer.

PPO PLAN

PATIENT INFO:

The patient is a 26 year old male who hurt his lower back helping his sister move four days ago. He is seeing the doctor today because the pain has increased, becoming more severe. He has been unable to work for the last 3 days. The patient has health insurance through his work. He has a PPO plan, no secondary plan and he is currently eligible for coverage.

PLAN INFO:

IN NETWORK:

No Deductible

80/20

$1000.00 Out of Pocket
($0.00 met to date)

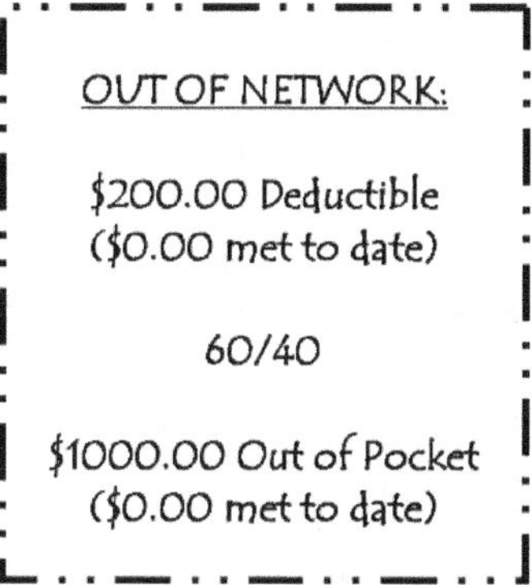

GENERAL INFO:

The doctor performed a new patient, problem-focused exam ($200.00), lower back X-Ray ($150.00) and wrote two prescriptions for medications. Total $350.00. The provider is in network and the allowed amount is the same as billed.

NOTES:

Expectations

Was the patient required to be seen by his PCP first?

- ☐ Yes
- ☐ No

Is a referral required?

- ☐ Yes
- ☐ No

What is the patient required to pay upfront?

- ☐ Zero
- ☐ $200.00
- ☐ $230.00
- ☐ $260.00
- ☐ $70.00
- ☐ $140.00

What is the health carrier expected to pay?

- ☐ Zero
- ☐ $280.00
- ☐ $210.00
- ☐ $70.00
- ☐ $140.00

The amount that the doctor is paid for his services is based on?

- ☐ The billed charges
- ☐ Contracted rates
- ☐ Usual, Customary and Reasonable

If the allowed amount is less than bill, how is the balance handled?

- ☐ Write off in full
- ☐ Patient responsibility

See the answer beginning on page 372

Case Study 3

Directions: Read the scenario below and answer any questions that follow. State your reasoning and any evidence to back up you answer.

THE CASE OF THE SILENT PROVISION

Jonas Wright is an avid skier and cyclist. So when he started to experience some back pain, he immediately called his doctor and set up an appointment because he did not want anything to interfere with the activities that he loved. The doctor felt that he could benefit from the services of a chiropractor. So Jonas consulted his plan booklet and was happy to learn that his plan provided unlimited in network and out of network chiropractic visits. Jonas was able to locate an out of network chiropractor that was close to his home with a reputation for providing excellent care. Jonas felt that their reputation alone justified him paying the higher out of network costs.

After he had incurred 12 visits, his Chiropractor called him to cancel all remaining scheduled visits citing that his plan does not pay for more than 5 chiropractic visits. Jonas immediately contacted his health carrier for clarification and again they confirmed that his plan provides unlimited visits and that all claims would be reprocessed. Shortly after, all of Jonas' claims were once again re-denied citing no coverage for out of network services beyond the 5 visits.

Jonas contacted a friend who did a three way conference call with Jonas and the insurance carrier and they learned that his plan has a "provision" that limited out of network chiropractic coverage to 5 visits. He could continue his care, only if he switched to an in network provider. So what is going on here? Does Jonas have a basis to dispute this requirement?

See the answer beginning on page 373

Case Study 4

Directions: Examine the information provided below and answer the questions that follow. Use what you have learned about plan types to help you arrive at your answer.

MEDICARE PLAN

PATIENT INFO: The patient is an 82 year old female. Other than her controlled high blood pressure, she is in good health. She is seeing the doctor today for her yearly blood pressure checkup with lab work and medication refills. Pt has Medicare and a Medigap plan.

PLAN INFO:

Medicare plan: $150.00 deductible ($0.00 met to date)

80/20 plan

Medigap plan: $150.00 deductible ($0.00 met to date) 20% of Medicare allowed.

GENERAL INFO: Established patient, problem-focused exam ($200.00), CBC ($75.00) and medication refill. Total $275.00. The provider participates with Medicare.

Note: Per the Medicare fee schedule, the allowed amount is $275.00

NOTES:

Expectations

Medicare is a plan for:

- ☐ Anyone, at any age.
- ☐ Low-income families with children, low-income elderly, and disabled people.
- ☐ 65 or older and younger people with disabilities or end stage renal disease.

Medigap is a plan for:

- ☐ Medicare beneficaries with tradional Medicare coverage only
- ☐ Those contracting with an out of network provider to provide service at in network rates.

Is a referral required?

- ☐ Yes
- ☐ No

What is the patient required to pay upfront?

- ☐ Zero
- ☐ $150.00 deductible only
- ☐ $175.00
- ☐ $275.00

What is Medicare expected to pay?

- ☐ Zero
- ☐ $100.00
- ☐ $220.00

What is Medigap expected to pay?

- ☐ Zero
- ☐ $25.00
- ☐ $125.00

See the answer on page 374

Case Study 5

Directions: Read the scenario below and answer any questions that follow. State your reasoning and any evidence to back up you answer.

THE CASE OF THE 'BUT I WANT ONE NOW!'

Mary Smith has Medicare as her primary plan and AARP as a secondary plan. Because a friend of hers just had a heart attack, she is concerned about her own health.

She goes to see her doctor and requests an EKG. The doctor listens to her heart, lists her overall chief complaints and symptoms, reviews her past history and tells Mary that her heart appears fine and that an EKG is just not necessary.

But Mary insists that she wants one now.

Since Mary has had Medicare for more than 12 months, this EKG will not qualify under the 'New to Medicare' visit. After much persistence, the doctor finally agrees to perform the EKG just to ease her anxiety.

Before the procedure is started, Mary is told that that the EKG may not be paid for by Medicare or her secondary plan because it may be deemed 'not medically necessary.' Mary understands and even agrees to pay the full price of $800.00 upfront. She feels that this money is well spent if it gives her the peace of mind she is seeking.

Mary's heart is good and the claim is billed to Medicare who denies the claim as not 'medically necessary.'

Mary calls the doctor's office shortly after receiving the denial and states that she was unaware that Medicare would not pay such a large bill. She lives on a fixed income and she just cannot afford to be out of pocket $800.00.

She requests a full refund.

Is the doctor's office required to refund her for a service that she asked for, paid for and agreed to in spite of being told in advance that it may not be covered?

See the answer beginning on page 374

Case Study 6

Directions: Examine the information provided below and answer the questions that follow. Use what you have learned about plan types to help you arrive at your answer.

FFS PLAN

PATIENT INFO: The patient is a 44 year old female who is in the office today due to a laceration to the hand. She cut her hand on broken glass washing dishes. The patient has health insurance through her work. She has an FFS plan, no secondary plan and is currently eligible for coverage.

PLAN INFO:

OUT OF NETWORK

$300.00 deductible ($300.00 met to date)

80/20 plan

$3000.00 Out of Pocket ($2800.00 met to date)

GENERAL INFO: Doctor performed an exam ($200.00) and laceration repair of the right palm with sutures ($350.00). Total $550.00. The allowed amount is $100.00 for the exam and $250.00 for the surgery.

NOTES:

Expectations

Is a referral required?

- ☐ Yes
- ☐ No

What is the patient required to pay upfront?

- ☐ Zero
- ☐ $70.00
- ☐ $200.00
- ☐ $270.00
- ☐ $550.00

What is the health carrier expected to pay?

- ☐ Zero
- ☐ $280.00
- ☐ $300.00
- ☐ $350.00
- ☐ $550.00

The amount that the doctor is paid for his services is based on?

- ☐ The billed charges
- ☐ Contracted rates
- ☐ Usual, Customary and Reasonable

If the allowed amount is less than the bill, how is the balance handled?

- ☐ Write off in full
- ☐ Patient responsibility

See the answer on page 375

Case Study 7

Directions: Read the scenario below and answer any questions that follow. State your reasoning and any evidence to back up you answer.

THE CASE OF THE 'ALL UP IN MY BUSINESS.'

Daphne G. is sitting in the triage room at her doctor's office. She has just explained to the nurse the reason for her visit, including: current complaints, medications and past history. She has also had her vitals checked. While waiting for a treatment room to become available, she overhears the nurse and a male patient talking in the next room. During the course of the exchange, she learns that the patient has a history of anxiety and diabetes and he is on medication for both. He is seeing the doctor today for a large ulcer on his right foot that has been slow to heal.

Because Daphne was able to hear so much of the conversation, she realizes that someone may have overheard all of her business as well. She complains to her doctor because she is concerned that her HIPAA rights were violated. Is she right?

See the answer on page 376

Case Study 8

Directions: Examine the information provided below and answer the questions that follow. Use what you have learned about plan types to help you arrive at your answer.

HMO PLAN

PATIENT INFO:

The patient is a 72 year old male patient with COPD. He is having problems getting around and he is in need of a power wheel chair. He arrived today at The Power Company to pick up his wheelchair.

PLAN INFO:

HMO plan: No deductible w/ 100% in network coverage only.

No out of network coverage

CLAIM PROCESSING INFO:

Power wheelchair to be provided by an outside vendor, The Power Company. The invoice price was negotiated from $2500.00 to $1800.00. Pt to arrange for pickup.

NOTES:

Expectations

Is pre-approval required?

- ☐ Yes
- ☐ No

Is a referral required?

- ☐ Yes
- ☐ No

What is the patient required to pay toward the cost of the wheelchair?

- ☐ Zero
- ☐ $700.00
- ☐ $1800.00
- ☐ $2500.00

What is the HMO plan expected to pay?

- ☐ Zero
- ☐ $1800.00
- ☐ $2500.00

How is the balance to be handled?

- ☐ Write off in full
- ☐ Patient responsibility

See the answer on page 376

Case Study 9

Directions: Read the scenario below and answer any questions that follow. State your reasoning and any evidence to back up you answer.

THE CASE OF THE INDIAN GIVER

Miles was in an auto accident two years ago. He was rear ended by a distracted driver and he suffered a head injury, a few broken bones and various soft tissue injuries. He has had numerous doctor visits, labs, x-rays, physical therapy, chiropractic therapy and lots of medications to help him recover. Thank goodness he has good health insurance coverage because he would not have been able to afford the thousands of dollars in health care expenses that he incurred.

He filed a lawsuit against the driver and his case was finally settled. He is dismayed to see that a large chunk of his settlement went to his health insurance carrier to reimburse them for paying all of his medical bills. Isn't that why he has health insurance in the first place, to pay for medical expenses? Can they just take back every dime that they paid?

See the answer on page 377

Case Study 10

Directions: Examine the information provided below and answer the questions that follow. Use what you have learned about plan types to help you arrive at your answer.

Individual and Family Deductible & Out of Pocket Maximum (OPE)

PATIENT INFO:

A family of 4 is being seen today by the family doctor that has treated them for years. They were involved in a motor vehicle accident earlier today but they declined transport to a local hospital because of the high emergency room costs. They have opted, instead, to see their own doctor for treatment. All injuries appeared to be non-life threatening.

PLAN INFO:

PPO

80/20 plan

$100.00 Individual Deductible
$300.00 Family Deductible

$1000.00 Individual OPE
$3000.00 Family OPE

This the first claims of the year for this family

GENERAL INFO: **PT 1 Adult** - Detailed Exam ($300.00), CT scan head/neck/shoulder ($3100.00), minor repair head laceration ($1800.00). Total = $5200.00

Pt 2 Adult - Detailed Exam ($300.00), CT Scan head/neck/leg ($2100.00), cast on left leg ($490.00). Total = $2890.00

Pt 3 Child - Detailed Exam ($300.00), X-ray shoulder/arm ($1200.00), cast left arm ($490.00), minor repair lacerations on left cheek, left arm and left knee ($3100.00). Total = $5090.00

Pt 4 Child in car seat - no injuries – Detailed Exam ($200.00). Total = $200.00

Provider is in network and allowed amounts are the same as billed. None of the patient or family deductible or OPE had been met prior to the accident.

CLAIM PROCESSING INFO:

All four claims were received on the same day but they were processed one after the other.

Pt. 1 was processed first
Pt. 4 was processed second
Pt. 3 was processed third
Pt. 2 was processed last

NOTES:

Expectations

PATIENT 1 (P1)

Will P1 meet his individual deductible when this claim is processed?

- ☐ Yes
- ☐ No

Will P1 meet his individual OPE when this claim is processed?

- ☐ Yes
- ☐ No

What was P1 required to pay on this claim?

- ☐ Zero
- ☐ $1120.00
- ☐ $1100.00
- ☐ $4080.00

What did the health carrier pay on this claim?

- ☐ Zero
- ☐ $80.00
- ☐ $4100.00
- ☐ $4080.00

PATIENT 4 (P4)

Will P4 meet her individual deductible when this claim is processed?

- ☐ Yes
- ☐ No

Will the family deductible be met when this claim sis processed?

- ☐ Yes

- ☐ No

What did P4 pay on this claim?

- ☐ Zero
- ☐ $100.00
- ☐ $120.00
- ☐ $200.00

What did the health carrier pay on this claim?

- ☐ Zero
- ☐ $80.00
- ☐ $100.00
- ☐ $200.00

PATIENT 3 (P3)

Will P3 meet his individual deductible when this claim is processed?

- ☐ Yes
- ☐ No

Will the family deductible met when this claim is processed?

- ☐ Yes
- ☐ No

What did P3 pay on this claim?

- ☐ Zero
- ☐ $1098.00
- ☐ $3990.00
- ☐ $5090.00

What did the health carrier pay on this claim?

- ☐ Zero
- ☐ $3992.00

- [ ] $3092.00
- [ ] $4072.00

Will P3 meet his individual OPE when the claim is processed?

- [ ] Yes
- [ ] No

PATIENT 2 (P2)

What did P2 pay on this claim?

- [ ] Zero
- [ ] $558.00
- [ ] $578.00
- [ ] $2890.00

What did the health carrier pay on this claim?

- [ ] Zero
- [ ] $2232.00
- [ ] $2312.00
- [ ] $2890.00

How much more is needed to satisify the family OPE for the year?

- [ ] Zero
- [ ] $84.00
- [ ] $104.00
- [ ] $404.00

See the answer beginning on page 377

Case Study 11

Directions: Read the scenario below and answer any questions that follow. State your reasoning and any evidence to back up you answer.

THE CASE OF THE MOBILE CHECKUP

Daniel had just pulled into the supermarket and stepped out of his car only to be approached by an attractive young lady who asked him if he wanted to have a no cost, full health screening designed to rule out all kinds of illnesses and diseases- from high blood pressure and cancer to diabetes and heart disease. He would not be charged a dime. His health plan would be billed and they would accept whatever his health carrier paid as payment in full. Daniel is in great health, with no current complaints but because he has a family history of health disease, he decides to go for it.

In the parking lot, a mini office/lab was set up on wheels. Daniel was asked to provide a copy of his health carrier ID card, given a form with a series of questions to answer and had some blood taken. He was told he would be notified by mail if they discovered anything. He was shocked to learn that his health plan had received a bill for $4200.00 for numerous lab tests and interpretation fees. It was hard to believe that they were able to perform so many tests with that one small vial of blood. His health carrier denied the full bill as not medical necessary. Was his health carrier justified in denying all of his tests?

See the answer on page 379

Case Study 12

Directions: Examine the information provided below and answer the questions that follow. Use what you have learned about plan types to help you arrive at your answer.

Coordination of Benefits COB

PATIENT INFO:

The patient is a 10 year old female that is being seen today for left leg pain. Patient was turning flips in the yard and landed on a sprinkler in the grass. She is unable to bear weight on the leg. Pt has two insurance plans, one from each of her parents who both have coverage through their jobs. The child resides with both parents.

PLAN INFO:

PLAN ONE:
Dad-Date of Birth 11/24/1980
PPO
$100.00 Deductible
($0.00 met to date)
80/20 plan
Preapproval for all services over $300.00

PLAN TWO:
Mom-Date of Birth 9/23/1980
HMO
$0.00 Deductible (In Network Only)
100% (In Network Only)
$10.00 Copay

GENERAL INFO:

Established patient, problem focused exam ($200.00), leg x-ray ($150.00), cast ($150.00). Total = $500.00. The provider is out of network with the PPO and in network with the HMO.

Note: The allowed amount is $500.00

NOTES:

Expectations

Is a referral required?

- ☐ Both the HMO and PPO
- ☐ Only the HMO
- ☐ Only the PPO
- ☐ Neither plans

Is pre-approval required?

- ☐ Both the HMO and PPO
- ☐ Only the HMO
- ☐ Only the PPO
- ☐ Neither plans

Which plan is primary?

- ☐ Mom's plan
- ☐ Dads plan

Determining who is prime is based on?

- ☐ Birthday rule
- ☐ Which parent is older
- ☐ Gender rule
- ☐ Who has custody

What is the patient required to pay upfront?

- ☐ Zero
- ☐ $10.00
- ☐ $150.00 deductible only
- ☐ $180.00

What is the HMO expected to pay?

- ☐ Zero

- [ ] $100.00
- [ ] $220.00
- [ ] $500.00

What is PPO expected to pay?

- [ ] Zero
- [ ] $320.00
- [ ] $400.00
- [ ] $500.00

See the answer beginning on page 379

Case Study 13

Directions: Read the scenario below and answer any questions that follow. State your reasoning and any evidence to back up you answer.

THE CASE OF THE CHECK IS IN THE MAIL

Raymond is 6 years old and has some health issues that has left him with severe weakness in his legs. He is eligible for a wheelchair, it is ordered and is shipped to his grandmother's house because she lives locally, and the dad is to pick it up after it arrives. His health plan is billed and they issue a payment to the father who is the plan holder.

The wheelchair company learns that payment had been issued, they obtain a copy of the check and it confirms that the check was signed and cashed by the dad, who continues to insist that the check was never received. Frustrated, the wheelchair company contacts the grandmother and learns that the chair had never been picked up by the father. They immediately send a truck, pick up the wheel chair and submit a corrected claim to the health plan asking them to void the claim and retrieve the payment that they made.

In the meantime, because the child has missed quite a few days from school due to his inability to get around, the school, unable to get the parents involved, contact Child Protective Services who open an investigation. They chastise the health insurance carrier for what they understand to be the problem which was their failure to provide the needed wheelchair. The health carrier issues a second check, this time payable to the wheel chair company. The wheel chair is delivered and the child is now mobile. The health insurance carrier, who is still out of pocket for the first payment, goes after the dad for reimbursement.

So how did this mess occur in the first place? What should the health carrier have done first?

See the answer on page 380

Case Study 14

Directions: Examine the information provided below and answer the questions that follow. Use what you have learned about plan types to help you arrive at your answer.

MEDICAID

PATIENT INFO: The patient is a 6 day old baby boy with some yellowing of the skin and the parents are concerned about jaundice. He is seeing the doctor today for blood work and a new patient exam. Pt has Medicaid only.

PLAN INFO:

Medicaid Traditional Plan

GENERAL INFO: New patient, problem-focused exam ($175.00), lab work ($100.00). Total $270.00. The provider participates with Medicaid in this state.

Note: Per the Medicaid Fee Schedule the allowed amount is $52.00 for the exam and $22.00 for the lab work. Total = $74.00

NOTES:

Expectations

Medicaid is a plan for:

- ☐ Low-income families with children, low-income elderly, and disabled people.
- ☐ 65 or older and younger people with disabilities or end stage renal disease.

Since provider participates with Medicaid in his state, he can:

- ☐ Refer this patient to another provider because of the low reimbursement.
- ☐ Treat this patient and have them pay in full.
- ☐ Treat the patient and bill Medicaid as he would any other health carrier.

Is a referral required:

- ☐ Yes
- ☐ No

What is the patient required to pay upfront:

- ☐ Zero
- ☐ $74.00
- ☐ $200.00
- ☐ $270.00

What is the Medicaid expected to pay:

- ☐ Zero
- ☐ $74.00
- ☐ $100.00
- ☐ $200.00

Any remaining balance is:

- ☐ The patients responsibility
- ☐ Will be adjusted off

See the answer beginning on page 381

Case Study 15

Directions: Read the scenario below and answer any questions that follow. State your reasoning and any evidence to back up you answer.

THE CASE OF THE EPIC FAIL

Jim is recently out of school and is excited about his new job as a Medical Biller for a General Practitioner. Jim has plenty of work to keep him busy but he is amazed at how easy it all is; create the claim, hit the submit button, upload the batch then start over. About 45 days later, the doctor he works for expresses concern about the lower volume of insurance payments that they are receiving. Jim gets on the phone to check status and learns that a lot of his claims were never received.

Jim doesn't understand. How can an electronic claim not be received?

See the answer on page 382

Case Study 16

Directions: Examine the information provided below and answer the questions that follow. Use what you have learned about plan types to help you arrive at your answer.

EPO PLAN

PATIENT INFO: The patient is a 16 year old male who fell off of his skateboard and injured his right arm and right shoulder. Pt denies hitting his head. Pt is being seen by Urgent Care for an evaluation and X-ray. Pt has a EPO plan only. No other coverage. Because parents consider this an emergency they take him to a center located just down the street. The provider nor the parents contacted the health plan for preapproval.

PLAN INFO:

EPO Plan: No deductible w/ 100% in network coverage only

No out of network coverage

GENERAL INFO: New patient, problem-focused exam ($300.00), arm and shoulder x-rays ($350.00). Cast of right arm ($100.00). Total $750.00 The provider is out of network.

NOTES:

Expectations

Is a referral or pre approval required?

- ☐ Yes
- ☐ No
- ☐ Waived in an emergency.

What is the patient required to pay upfront?

- ☐ Zero
- ☐ $750.00

What is the EPO plan expected to pay?

- ☐ Zero
- ☐ $750.00

If the allowed amount is less than the bill, how is the balance handled?

- ☐ Write off in full
- ☐ Patient responsibility

If the patient was admitted to an out of network hospital for his injuries and approval was granted in advance, what is the EPO plan expected to pay for this portion of the bill?

- ☐ Zero
- ☐ 100% of allowed amount.

See the answer beginning on page 382

Case Study 17

Directions: Read the scenario below and answer any questions that follow. State your reasoning and any evidence to back up you answer.

THE CASE OF THE ONE MONKEY STOPS THE SHOW

Beverly and her husband are covered under an EPO health plan though her place of employment. Her premium payments are high but they are deducted from her check every two weeks without fail. Besides, her health coverage is great. Beverly's husband injures his knee playing golf and while visiting the doctor she is asked to pay for the visit in full because her plan is showing that she is no longer eligible for coverage. Beverly assures the doctor's office that her premium is paid and she even shows them her pay stub showing the recent premium deduction. The doctor's office and Beverly get on a three way call with the health carrier and learn that the premium is lapse. "Not possible," says Beverly. She has been paying all of her premiums every month, on time. She is unable to get the health carrier to budge so she pulls out her credit card and pays for the visit in full. She is extremely upset and vows to report the bad service to her employer. What could be going on here? Is her health carrier at fault here?

See the answer beginning on page 382

Case Study 18

Directions: Examine the information provided below and answer the questions that follow. Use what you have learned about plan types to help you arrive at your answer.

POS PLAN

PATIENT INFO:

33 year old patient is currently seeing three different providers, an HMO provider for treatment of her high blood pressure, an in network PPO chiropractor for back pain and an out of network dermatologist.

PLAN INFO:

HMO	PPO	OUT OF NETWORK
No Deductible	$100.00 Deductible ($0.00 met to date)	$500.00 Deductible ($0.00 met to date)
$10.00 Copay	80/20 Plan	60/40 Plan
100% In Network	$500.00 OPE ($0.00 met to date)	$1000.00 OPE ($0.00 met to date)

GENERAL INFO: HMO provider - Detailed exam ($150.00) and bloodwork ($150.00). Total = $300.00.

Chiropractor - Weekly therapy visit ($200.00). Total = $200.00

Dermatologist - Weekly treatment of Acne ($150.00). Total = $150.00

Billed amount is the same as allowed.

NOTES:

Expectations

Is a referral required for the Chiropratice or Dermatologist visits?

- ☐ Yes
- ☐ No

What is the patient required to pay to the HMO provider?

- ☐ Zero
- ☐ $10.00
- ☐ $58.00
- ☐ 290.00

What is the health carrier expected to pay to the HMO provider?

- ☐ Zero
- ☐ $232.00
- ☐ $290.00
- ☐ $300.00

What is the patient required to pay to the Chiropractor?

- ☐ Zero
- ☐ $10.00
- ☐ $120.00
- ☐ 200.00

What is the health carrier expected to pay to the Chiropractor?

- ☐ Zero
- ☐ $80.00
- ☐ $160.00
- ☐ $200.00

What is the patient expected to pay to the Dermatologist?

- ☐ Zero
- ☐ $10.00
- ☐ $60.00
- ☐ $150.00

What is the health carrier expected to pay to the Dermatologist?

- ☐ Zero
- ☐ $90.00
- ☐ $120.00
- ☐ $150.00

See the answer beginning on page 383

Case Study 19

Directions: Read the scenario below and answer any questions that follow. State your reasoning and any evidence to back up you answer.

THE CASE OF THE NEVER CAN SAY GOODBYE

Daisy is 65 years old, retired and finally eligible for Medicare. She knows that her current doctor participates with traditional Medicare but her son encourages her to switch to a Medicare HMO plan, which is a managed care plan, because it will be so much better for her due to its wide range of doctors under one network as well as the fact she will only have to pay a $20.00 per visit copay.

She is not happy with having to leave the doctor that has treated her for the last 14 years. In spite of her misgivings, she switches and immediately hates the new plan. She wants to go back to her old doctor.

Can Daisy just switch back after she has enrolled?

See the answer on page 384

Case Study 20

Directions: Examine the information provided below and answer the questions that follow. Use what you have learned about plan types to help you arrive at your answer.

Account Reconciliation

PATIENT INFO: The patient is a 35 year old female who was seen in the office 6 weeks ago for fever, bilateral ear pain, sore throat and cough. Pt requested a chest X-ray, but chest sounds were clear so she was advised by the doctor that the chest X-ray may not be covered by her health plan. She understands but wants it anyway. Patient has two plans. Total claim billed $890.00

PLAN INFO:

<u>PLAN ONE</u>

Effective 01/01/2015
PPO
$100.00 Deductible
($55.00 met to date)
80/20 Plan
$1000.00 OPE
($0.00 met to date)

<u>PLAN TWO</u>

Effective 01/01/2014
Medicaid
100%
$0.00 Deductible

GENERAL INFO:

<u>Primary Plan EOB</u>

Billed: $890.00
Allowed: $555.00
Denied: $80.00 chest X-ray not covered

<u>Secondary Plan EOB</u>

Billed $890.00
Allowed: $525.00
Denied: $80.00 chest X-ray not covered

Provider participates with both plans

The Medical Biller received 2 payments in the mail today, one from the PPO plan and another payment from the Medicaid plan.

Expectations

Which plan is primary, which is secondary?

- ☐ The PPO plan is prime and the Medicaid is secondary
- ☐ The Medicaid Plan is primary and the PPO is secondary

What did the primary carrier pay for this visit?

- ☐ Zero
- ☐ $408.00
- ☐ $612.00
- ☐ $890.00

What did the secondary plan pay?

- ☐ Zero
- ☐ $30.00
- ☐ $117.00
- ☐ $335.00

What did the patient pay for this visit?

- ☐ Zero
- ☐ $45.00
- ☐ $80.00
- ☐ $102.00
- ☐ $227.00

Was the patient required to sign a ABN before the chest x-ray was taken?

- ☐ Yes
- ☐ No

Why was the chest x-ray not covered?

- ☐ No referral was in place
- ☐ No pre approval was in place
- ☐ The service was not medically necessary

The $80.00 charge for the chest X-ray…

- ☐ Must be written off to the patient since she has Medicaid
- ☐ Can be billed to the patient
- ☐ Must be adjusted off since both providers are participating.

Any other charges that were not allowed will be?

- ☐ Written off
- ☐ Billed to the patient

Was the Individual deductible met on this claim?

- ☐ Yes
- ☐ No

How much of the OPE was met on this claim?

- ☐ Zero
- ☐ $30.00
- ☐ $80.00
- ☐ $102.00

See the answer beginning on page 384

SOLUTIONS

CHAPTER 1 TEST SOLUTIONS

1. The purpose of the ACA was twofold; to provide access to health care to the millions of uninsured Americans and to reduce government spending.
2. Universal Healthcare is coverage provided to all citizens to a particular country. The ACA does not provide coverage to all citizens. Coverage is based on eligibility and one's ability to pay.
3. To have better visibility into the overall health of the plan and to help control healthcare costs.
4. ERISA's role is to protect plan members covered under employer sponsored plans. This ensures accountability, transparency and clarity from premium collection to claim filing to appeals.
5. Credible coverage is prior health coverage that was under a group, individual, Medicare, Medicaid, Tricare, Indian Health, state high risk or federal plan.
6. The employer.
7. No. Fully insured plans are administered by health insurance carriers who are in the business of handling all aspects of claims processing.
8. Administrative Services Only.
9. A Business Associate Agreement is a legal agreement that details how shared protected health information should be kept secure.
10. With Group plans, the risk and premiums are shared by all members of the group and on an individual plan the lone member bears the costs.
11. No. Even if this information is common knowledge, you do not have a "need to know" so you do not have a right to disclose.

CHAPTER 2 TEST SOLUTIONS

1. Yes, but the reimbursement levels will be lower than if they used an in network provider.
2. Use the very small network providers or pay out of pocket.
3. Per Member Per Month refers to the way providers are paid under HMO plans.
4. HMO plan.
5. A medical provider because they have the ability to bill any amount they choose and balance bill the patient what is not covered by the health plan.
6. Acompany that is in the business of writing and selling health plans.
7. Help control health care costs.
8. Spend down is the process of using medical expenses to help meet Medicaid eligibility.
9. When you are approaching age 65 you have 7 months to enroll in Medicare; 3 months before your birthday, the month of your birthday and 3 months after your birthday.
10. No

11. Champus
12. Health plans do not cover work related illness or injury so the claim may be denied if not authorized to treat.
13. BCBS ID numbers have Alpha prefix that make these easy to associated with BCBS.

CHAPTER 3 TEST SOLUTIONS

1. The timing of when a claim reaches the health carrier will affect how the deductible is applied. The deductible is taken from the first claim(s) received by the health carrier.
2. Family deductibles help to minimize the costs that families have to pay for healthcare.
3. Out of pocket refers to the amount that a patient is expected to pay for healthcare.
4. Cost sharing.
5. To have access to patients that are covered under managed care plans.
6. Access to patients covered under managed care plans may not be enough to justify the lower reimbursement rates.
7. Act as a gatekeeper by managing a patient's access to care.
8. No. Call and confirm on all new patients.
9. UR's role is to direct patients to the best level of care in order to help control costs.
10. If you believe that you will have to go more than 63 days without health care.
11. A specialist or out of network services, treatments or supplies
12. As a way to facilitate access to care at a pre-negotiated cost or benefit.
13. False

CHAPTER 4 TEST SOLUTIONS

1. Coding is the process of selecting the appropriate codes to accurately describe the reason for the visit as well as all treatments and services that was performed. Billing is the process of taking those same codes to create and submit a claim for reimbursement.
2. If a valid code is not available, a miscellaneous code should be used along with a written report that describes what services were performed.
3. ICD-10 is used to report a patient's diagnosis, symptoms or condition and a CPT-4 code is used to describe all services, treatments and supplies that were performed.
4. The CPT-4 Manual
5. The ICD-9 codes are used for all dates of service prior to 10/1/15.
6. A HCPCS Level I code is used when billing Medicare and Medicaid. HCPCS Level II codes are used to bill for non-physician related services like ambulance, drugs, DME etc.
7. NPI. They are used most often and are required by all health carriers for billing, claim inquiry and disputes.
8. 24B.

9. Since the CMS 1500 leaves little room for documentation, a modifier is used to further explain clarify, alter or add to a patient's encounter.
10. Coding to the highest level of specificity means coding all that you know to be true and confirmed about a patient's condition.

CHAPTER 5 TEST SOLUTIONS

1. Clean claim means that the claim has everything it needs to get processed at first submission. This includes correct patient, plan and provider information as well as all supported codes and modifiers.
2. AOB refers to the Assignments of Benefits form that is used to designate who should receive claim payments; the patient or the provider.
3. Box 13 is the assignment field on a CMS 1500 form. A live signature or SOF (signature on file) tells the health carrier to pay the provider directly, if left blank it tells the carrier to pay the patient.
4. ***Scrub the claim*** refers to the process that a clearinghouse uses to check for errors and edits before sending the claim on the health carrier for processing.
5. COB - Coordination of Benefits is the process of determining which health carrier to bill first, second and even third when a patient has more than one health insurance plan.
6. In network providers are normally paid directly, unless a patient can support that the claim was paid, in full, at time of service.
7. A batch file is simply a folder of all claims that are ready to be submitted on to the clearinghouse after being created by the biller.
8. HIPAA has implemented requirements for protection of a patient's health information. All Clearinghouses are required to adhere to these HIPAA standards when transmitting data.
9. The Release of Information form gives permission for a patient's personal information to be released for the purpose of claim billing and claim processing.
10. Not likely. It is not a patient's fault if a biller fails to keep track and submit claims within the timely filing period.

CHAPTER 6 TEST SOLUTIONS

1. Answers will vary.
2. Answers will vary.

An example is:

Understanding the journey is eye opening, as it helps you to understand the many hands that will touch that claim, for a multitude of different reasons; from first encounter to final processing. Understanding the process helps you to understand what frontend steps must be taken to ensure the desired outcome.

CHAPTER 7 TEST SOLUTIONS

A	Contracted rate	**F**	The amount the provider is required to adjust off a patient's account.
B	UCR	**E**	The electronic transfer of claim payments.
C	Allowed amount	**G**	A statement that shows how a claim was processed.
D	Fee schedule	**A**	Reimbursement rate that is agreed to, by contract, between a participating provider and the health carrier.
E	EFT	**H**	Contacting the health carrier to dispute the way a claim was processed.
F	Write off	**B**	The usual or average charge for a service, treatment, or supply.
G	EOB	**C**	The portion of the billed charges that is covered by the plan.
H	Appeal	**I**	The process of keeping ones eye on all aspects of a provider's practice to ensure that it is profitable.
I	Revenue Management	**D**	A list of the allowed amounts for each valid CPT code.

CHAPTER 8 TEST SOLUTIONS

1. Can the service be provided in network? And is the service medically necessary?
2. Pre-approval means that a service, treatment or supply has been deemed to be medically necessary but this approval does not mean that the patient's health plan provides coverage.
3. 4 levels
4. No. the process may differ by state, by carrier and by plan.
5. The reference number is a link to the diary of the call. What you initially called about? Who you spoke to? What was the promised resolution? Etc. This way if you have to call back about the same issue you will not have to repeat the same story.
6. Yes. Coverage, benefits and plan provisions change and patients oftentimes fail to provide the most accurate or the most current information. This could result in limited or no reimbursement. The verification process only takes a few minutes, better to safe than sorry.
7. No. The Benefit Booklet provides full benefits, provisions and limitations. You will only need to consult this booklet if a call to the health carrier fails to answer a question you have about a patient's coverage.
8. To obtain a list of the EOB/RA codes and descriptions that some health carriers use on their EOB/RA's
9. Version 2-12.
10. Medicare says that unless the service, treatment or supply is life threating or affects the safety of the patient if they refuse signature, the provider should refuse to treat.

CHAPTER 9 TEST SOLUTIONS

D	Credentialing	A	National Provider Identification Number.
J	Assignment	B	All of the various processes that a claim goes through once it reaches the health carrier that will result in the final disposition of that claim.
G	Limiting Charge	C	Breaking down a service, treatment, or supply into numerous different charges when it should have included, all together, as one charge.
H	Open Enrollment	D	The process of verifying and accepting a healthcare provider before they being allowed to participate as an in network provider.
F	Mandated Benefits	E	Medicare coverage for professional services
C	Unbundling	F	A type of benefit, provision or coverage that must be offered by law.
A	NPI	G	115% of the Medicare allowed amount is all that non-participating provider is allowed to charge a Medicare patient.
B	Adjudication	H	The period, normally once per year, where a plan member can switch from one plan to another, if offered.
E	Part B	I	Advance Beneficiary Notice
I	ABN	J	Permission to pay all claim payments directly to the provider of service.

C/S 1: THE CASE OF THE PREEXISTING CONDITION-SOLVED

The answer can be found in Chapter Three under the ***Cobra*** heading; under the heading "Why Enroll in Cobra."

In order not to be subject to a preexisting period, one must not lose coverage for more than 63 days. Because Ashton allowed three months, or 90 days, to elapse before he was enrolled in Sierra Social Services Agency's medical insurance, he was subject to the preexisting condition and therefore required to pay, out of his pocket, the $722.00 for his Dr.'s visit and labs incurred on July 15, 2014.

C/S 2: PPO PLAN-SOLVED

Was the patient required to be seen by his PCP first?

- ☐ Yes
- ✓ **No**

Is a referral required?

- ☐ Yes
- ✓ **No**

What is the patient required to pay upfront?

- ☐ Zero
- ☐ $200.00
- ☐ $230.00
- ☐ $260.00
- ✓ **$70.00 ($350.00 x 20%)**
- ☐ $140.00

What is the health carrier expected to pay?

- ☐ Zero
- ✓ **$280.00 ($350.00 x 80%)**
- ☐ $210.00
- ☐ $70.00
- ☐ $140.00

The amount that the doctor is paid for his services is based on?

- ☐ The billed charges
- ✓ **Contracted rates**
- ☐ Usual, Customary and Reasonable

If the allowed amount is less than bill, how is the balance handled?

- ✓ **Write off in full**
- ☐ Patient responsibility

C/S 3: THE CASE OF THE SILENT PROVISION-SOLVED

Yes, "Jonas" has a basis to dispute this requirement. Jonas did not want to change to another Chiropractor because he was feeling much better and was on his way to a full recovery. I suggested that he appeal based on Continuity of Care.

An appeal citing Continuity of Care simply means that we contact the health carrier and ask them to allow a continuation of the care that is being received with no disruptions or changes.

We submitted a written appeal explaining why a change to another Chiropractor would slow down his current process, may harm his health and could end up costing the plan more due to a possible increase in the number of visits needed to get him back to where he was before he was forced to change. We included his treatment plan and all documents that supported the fact that his condition had improved.

His health carrier reviewed his request and approved coverage for the same chiropractor until he was released from care.

C/S 4: MEDICARE PLAN-SOLVED

Medicare is a plan for:

- ☐ Anyone, at any age can enroll
- ☐ Low-income families with children, low-income elderly, and disabled people.
- ✓ **65 or older and younger people with disabilities or end stage renal disease.**

Medigap is a plan for:

- ✓ **Medicare beneficaries with tradional Medicare coverage only.**
- ☐ Contracting with an out of network provider to provide service at in network rates

Is a referral required?

- ☐ Yes
- ✓ **No**

What is the patient required to pay upfront?

- ☐ Zero
- ✓ **$150.00 deductible only (Both plans have an unsatisfied plan deductible)**
- ☐ $175.00
- ☐ $275.00

What is Medicare expected to pay?

- ☐ Zero
- ✓ **$100.00 ($275 - $150 (deductible) = $125.00 x 80%)**
- ☐ $220.00

What is Medigap expected to pay?

- ☐ Zero
- ✓ **$25.00 ($275 - $150 (deductible) = $125.00 x 20%)**
- ☐ $125.00

C/S 5: THE CASE OF 'BUT I WANT ONE NOW'-SOLVED

The answer can be found in Chapter 8 under the heading *How to Issue an ABN.*

The Center for Medicare and Medicaid Services (CMS) mandates that a Medicare Beneficiary must be advised, before services are rendered, that Medicare may deny coverage for a service or supply.

A CMS approved ABN form must be signed by the beneficiary as acknowledgement that they understand that the claim may not be covered, but they want to proceed with the service/supply anyway.

The patient cannot be held financially liable if a signed ABN is not obtained.

In this case, although the patient verbally agreed and then recanted, she cannot be held liable because an ABN was not sign. She is due a full refund.

C/S 6: FFS PLAN-SOLVED

Is a referral required?

- ☐ Yes
- ✓ **No**

What is the patient required to pay upfront?

- ☐ Zero
- ☐ $70.00
- ☐ $200.00
- ✓ **$270.00 ($350.00 x 20% = $70.00 + 200.00 over allowed)**
- ☐ $350.00
- ☐ $550.00

What is the health carrier expected to pay?

- ☐ Zero
- ✓ **$280.00 ($350.00 x 80%)**
- ☐ $350.00
- ☐ $550.00

The amount that the doctor is paid for his services is based on?

- ☐ The billed charges
- ☐ Contracted rates
- ✓ **Usual, Customary and Reasonable**

If the allowed amount is less than the bill, how is the balance handled?

- ☐ Write off in full
- ✓ **Patient responsibility**

C/S 7: THE CASE OF THE ALL UP IN MY BUSINESS-SOLVED

The answer can be found in Chapter 1, under the heading *HIPAA*.

No, not necessarily. Protected Health Information (PHI) is any and all information that you have or have access to about a person's past, current or future medical conditions both physical and mental OR any information that can be used to identify or link any type of treatment, services or diagnosis to a particular person including their name, address, date of birth, social security number, ID number, etc.

Since Daphne was not able to identify the male voice nor could anyone other than the nurse identify her, no breach of Protected Health Information (PHI) had occurred. HIPAA provides protection for a patient's past, current and future health conditions against disclosure to anyone that can link the condition and the patient together. That being said, I say "not necessarily," because had Daphne and the male patient walked out of the triage rooms at the same time and realized that they knew each other, a breach ***may*** have occurred.

C/S 8: HMO PLAN-SOLVED

Is pre-approval required?

- ✓ **Yes**
- ☐ No

Is a referral required?

- ✓ **Yes**
- ☐ No

What is the patient required to pay toward the cost of the wheelchair?

- ✓ **Zero (100% coverage price negotiated in advance)**
- ☐ $700.00
- ☐ $1800.00
- ☐ $2500.00

What is the HMO plan expected to pay?

- ☐ Zero
- ✓ **$1800.00 (Reimbursement price was negotiated in advance)**
- ☐ $2500.00

How is the balance to be handled?

- ✓ **Write off in full**
- ☐ Patient responsibility

C/S 9: THE CASE OF THE INDIAN GIVER-SOLVED

The answer can be found in Chapter 3, under the heading *Subrogation.*

If a health plan includes a subrogation clause, yes, they have the right to recover any amount that they paid due to a negligent third party. If your case settles and your health insurance carrier, based on the Subrogation Clause, is entitled to be reimbursed for all or a portion of what they paid out for the accident related medical expenses that were incurred, please believe they will collect. Most attorneys build this into the settlement.

C/S 10: INDIVID. & FAM. DEDUCTIBLE & OOP PLAN-SOLVED

PATIENT 1 (P1)

Will P1 meet his individual deductible when this claim is processed?

- ✓ **Yes**
- ☐ No

Will P1 meet his individual OPE when this claim is processed?

- ✓ **Yes**
- ☐ No

What was P1 required to pay on this claim?

- ☐ Zero
- ☐ $1040.00
- ✓ **$1100.00 ($100.00 deductible and $1000.00 OPE)**
- ☐ $4080.00

What did the health carrier pay on this claim?

- ☐ Zero
- ☐ $80.00
- ✓ **$4100.00 (Balance after pt. liability is met)**
- ☐ $4080.00

PATIENT 4 (P4)

Will P4 meet her individual deductible when this claim is processed?

- ✓ **Yes**
- ☐ No

Will the family deductible be met when this claim is processed?

- ☐ Yes
- ✓ **No**

What did P4 pay on this claim?

- ☐ Zero
- ☐ $100.00
- ✓ **$120.00 ($100.00 deductible + $100.00 x 20%)**
- ☐ $200.00

What did the health carrier pay on this claim?

- ☐ Zero
- ✓ **$80.00 ($100.00 x 80%)**
- ☐ $100.00
- ☐ $200.00

PATIENT 3 (P3)

Will P3 meet his individual deductible when this claim is processed?

- ✓ **Yes**
- ☐ No

Will the family deductible met when this claim is processed?

- ✓ **Yes**
- ☐ No

What did P3 pay on this claim?

- ☐ Zero
- ✓ **$1098.00 ($5090.00 – 100.00 deductible = $4999.00 x 20% + deductible)**
- ☐ $3990.00
- ☐ $5090.00

What did the health carrier pay on this claim?

- ☐ Zero
- ✓ **$3992.00 ($5090.00 – 100.00 deductible = $4990.00 x 80%)**
- ☐ $3092.00
- ☐ $4072.00

Will P3 meet his individual OPE when the claim is processed?

- ☐ Yes
- ✓ **No**

PATIENT 2 (P2)

What did P2 pay on this claim?

- ☐ Zero
- ☐ $558.00
- ✓ **$578.00 ($2890.00 x 20%)**
- ☐ $2890.00

What did the health carrier pay on this claim?

- ☐ Zero
- ☐ $2232.00
- ✓ **$2312.00 ($2890.00 x 80%)**
- ☐ $2890.00

How much more is needed to satisify the family OPE for the year?

- ☐ Zero
- ☐ $84.00
- ☐ $104.00
- ✓ **$404.00 ($3000.00 OPE - $2596.00 [P1 $1000.00 + P4 $20.00 + P3 $998.00 + P4 $578.00])**

C/S 11: THE CASE OF THE MOBILE CHECK UP-SOLVED

The answer can be found in Chapter 3, under the heading *Medical Necessity*.

Medical necessity means that there must be a reason in order to have any medical services performed. Just wanting to know, wishing to rule out a particular condition or simply needing to quiet your fears, does not qualify as medically necessary.

In this case, Daniel had no reason to see a doctor that day. He had no concerns about his health. In fact, he was on his way to the store. All of the tests that were performed were unnecessary and therefore not payable under the plan.

C/S 12: COB PLAN-SOLVED

Is a referral required?

- ☐ Both the HMO and PPO
- ☐ Only the HMO
- ☐ Only the PPO
- ✓ **Neither plans**

Is pre-approval required?

- ☐ Both the HMO and PPO

- ☐ Only the HMO
- ☐ Only the PPO
- ✓ **Neither plans (Because 100% was expected from the primary plan – preapproval was waived from the secondary carrier)**

Which plan is primary?

- ✓ **Mom's plan**
- ☐ Dads plan

Determining who is prime is based on?

- ✓ **Birthday rule**
- ☐ Which parent is older
- ☐ Gender rule
- ☐ Who has custody

What is the patient required to pay upfront?

- ☐ Zero
- ✓ **$10.00 (HMO copay)**
- ☐ $150.00 deductible only
- ☐ $180.00

What is the HMO expected to pay?

- ☐ Zero
- ☐ $100.00
- ☐ $220.00
- ✓ **$500.00 (100% of billed)**

What is PPO expected to pay?

- ✓ **Zero (paid in full by primary)**
- ☐ 320.00
- ☐ $400.00
- ☐ $500.00

C/S 13: THE CASE OF THE CHECK IS IN THE MAIL-SOLVED

The answer can be found in Chapter 5, under the heading *Assignment of Benefits.*

To solve the problem of not having the patient available when a claim needs to be billed, the provider's office will have the authorized person sign an Assignment of Benefits Form (AOB) when they are in the office. The problem occurred because the wheelchair company failed to have an AOB on file.

Because they did not get a signature from the parent authorizing payment go directly to the wheelchair company, they had to bill the claim as an unassigned claim. The check was issued to Dad who cashed it and refused to pay the wheelchair company. Not wanting to be at a loss, the wheelchair company took back the wheelchair and voided the claim leaving the child without one.

C/S 14: MEDICAID PLAN-SOLVED

Medicaid is a plan for?

- ✓ **Low-income families with children, low-income elderly, and disabled people.**
- ☐ 65 or older and younger people with disabilities or end stage renal disease.

The provider participates with Medicaid in this state, he can

- ☐ Refer this patient to another provider because of the low reimbursement.
- ☐ Treat this patient and have them pay in full.
- ✓ Treat the patient and bill Medicaid as he would any other health carrier.

Is a referral required?

- ☐ Yes
- ✓ **No**

What is the patient required to pay upfront?

- ✓ **Zero (Medicaid plan pays 100% of allowed)**
- ☐ $100.00
- ☐ $200.00
- ☐ $300.00

What is Medicaid expected to pay?

- ☐ Zero
- ✓ **$74.00 (100% of Medicaid allowed)**
- ☐ $100.00
- ☐ $200.00

Any remaining balance is?

- ☐ The patient's responsibility
- ✓ **Adjusted off**

C/S 15: THE CASE OF THE EPIC FAIL-SOLVED

The answer can be found in Chapter 5, under the heading *Clearinghouse,* under the heading "Claims with errors need to be fixed immediately."

Jim was not checking the clearinghouse for errors. If the claim is not corrected and resubmitted, it will remain in a holding pattern, unprocessed and aging until some human takes the time to review it. The health carrier will have no record of these claims because they would have been returned before they even reached the health carrier.

C/S 16: EPO PLAN-SOLVED

Is a referral or preapproval required?

- ✓ **Yes**
- ☐ No
- ☐ Waived in an emergency.

What is the patient required to pay upfront?

- ☐ Zero
- ✓ **$750.00 (out of network provider with no preapproval or referral)**

What is the EPO plan expected to pay?

- ✓ **Zero (non life threatening injuries treated by a non-approved out of network provider.)**
- ☐ $750.00

If the allowed amount is less than the bill, how is the balance handled?

- ☐ Write off in full
- ✓ **Patient responsibility**

If the patient was admitted to an out of network hospital for his injuries, what is the EPO plan expected to pay for this portion of the bill?

- ☐ Zero
- ✓ **Depends on if preapproval was obtained**
- ☐ 100% of allowed amount.

C/S 17: THE CASE OF ONE MONKEY STOPS THE SHOW-SOLVED

The answer can be found in Chapter 1, under the heading *Self-Funded Plan.*

Because Beverly had not bothered to read her plan booklet, she was not aware that her plan was self-funded. This means the employer must have the funds to pay all claims incurred by the group of employees. The monthly premium is a combined payment from the employer and all employees. The employees were paying their portion, by automatic deduction each pay period, but the employer was running short on funds so he was unable to come up with his share. Because this is group plan, if the premium is not paid in full, insurance coverage for all members of the group will lapse until brought current.

Outcome: The employer remedies the issue. Beverly was able to get reimbursed by her health carrier for the money she paid upfront for her husband's care.

C/S 18: POS PLAN-SOLVED

Is a referral required for the Chiropratice or Dermatologist visits?

- ☐ Yes
- ✓ **No**

What is the patient required to pay to the HMO provider?

- ☐ Zero
- ✓ **$10.00 (HMO copay only)**
- ☐ $58.00
- ☐ 290.00

What is the health carrier expected to pay to the HMO provider?

- ☐ Zero
- ☐ $232.00
- ☐ $290.00
- ✓ **$300.00 (100% of billed)**

What is the patient required to pay to the Chiroprator?

- ☐ Zero
- ☐ $10.00
- ✓ **$120.00 ($200 - $100 deductible = $100.00 x 20%)**
- ☐ 200.00

What is the health carrier expected to pay to the Chiroprator?

- ☐ Zero
- ✓ **$80.00 ($100.00 x 80%)**
- ☐ $160.00
- ☐ $200.00

What is the patient expected to pay to the Dermatologist?

- ☐ Zero
- ☐ $10.00

- ☐ $60.00
- ✓ **$150.00 (Deductible not met)**

What is the health carrier expected to pay to the Dermatologist?

- ✓ **Zero (Deductible not met)**
- ☐ $90.00
- ☐ $120.00
- ☐ $150.00

C/S 19: THE CASE OF THE NEVER CAN SAY GOODBYE-SOLVED

The answer can be found in Chapter 2, under the heading *Medicare*, under the WINK section.

During the first 45 days of coverage, Medicare beneficiaries can change from a Managed Care Plan to original (traditional) Medicare. So as long as 45 days has not passed, Daisy can switch back to the doctor she loves.

C/S 20: ACCOUNT RECONCILIATION PLAN-SOLVED

Which plan is primary, which is secondary?

- ✓ **The PPO plan is prime and the Medicaid is secondary**
- ☐ The Medicaid Plan is primary and the PPO is secondary

What did the Primary Carrier pay for this visit?

- ☐ Zero
- ✓ **$408.00 ($555.00 - $45.00 deductible = $510.00 x 80%)**
- ☐ $612.00
- ☐ $890.00

What did the secondary plan pay?

- ☐ Zero
- ☐ $30.00
- ✓ **$117.00 ($525.00 allowed - $408.00 (primary paid))**
- ☐ $335.00

What did the patient pay for this visit?

- ☐ Zero
- ☐ $45.00
- ✓ **$80.00 ($80.00 chest x-ray only. Provider received 100% of Medicaid allowed)**

- ☐ $102.00
- ☐ $125.00

Was the patient required to sign a ABN before the chest x-ray was taken?

- ☐ Yes
- ✓ **No**

Why was the chest x-ray not covered?

- ☐ No referral was in place
- ☐ No pre approval was in place
- ✓ **The service was not medically necessary**

The $80.00 charge for the chest X-ray…

- ☐ Must be written off to the patient since she has Medicaid
- ✓ **Can be billed to the patient**
- ☐ Must be adjusted off since both providers are participating.

Any other charges that were not allowed will be?

- ✓ **Written off**
- ☐ Billed to the patient

Was the Individual deductible met on this claim?

- ✓ **Yes**
- ☐ No

How much of the OPE was met on this claim?

- ✓ **Zero (100% of Medicaid allowed was paid, the chest x-ray does not apply to the OPE)**
- ☐ $30.00
- ☐ $80.00
- ☐ $102.00

REFERENCES

We would be remiss if we didn't give credit to those who helped us with accurately conveying certain facts, figures, dates, years, and otherwise other vital statistics crucial to the completion of the *1500pays: A Health Insurance Guide.* Our purpose was meant to expose you to the practical side of medical billing-what you will experience on the day-to-day. We encourage all of our readers to visit these sites and view these wonderful resources in depth if you find yourself interested in the informational side of any of the articles presented in this guide.

These Sources Include:

www.hhs.gov

www.dol.gov

www.hbma.org

www.palmettogba.com

www.tricare.mil

www.cdc.gov

www.cms.gov

www.wikipedia.org

References In Order of Appearance

ACA (*Key changes by year*)

Key Features of the Affordable Care Act By Year | HHS.gov. (n.d.). Retrieved October 21, 2016, from http://www.hhs.gov/healthcare/facts-and-features/key-features-of-aca-by-year/index.html

Universal Care (*Countries with some form of Universal Healthcare*)

Universal health care countries list, Search.com. (n.d.). Retrieved October 21, 2016, from https://www.search.com/web/universal-health-care-countries-list

ERISA (*Important ERISA Protections*)

Health Plans & Benefits | United States Department of Labor. (n.d.). Retrieved October 21, 2016, from http://www.dol.gov/general/topic/health-plans

HIPAA (Titles/PHI/Business Associate Agreement)

Health Insurance Portability and Accountability Act ... (n.d.). Retrieved October 21, 2016, from https://en.wikipedia.org/wiki/Health_Insurance_Portability_and_Accountability_Act

Railroad Medicare (Prefix descriptions)

JM Part A. (n.d.). Retrieved October 26, 2016, from http://www.palmettogba.com/Palmetto/Providers.Nsf/DocsCatHome/JM Part A

Military (Plan Types, Categories, Restructuring)

Health Plans | TRICARE. (n.d.). Retrieved October 21, 2016, from http://www.tricare.mil/Plans/HealthPlans

CPT-4 Codes (*CPT-4 Codes fall into 3 categories*)

Current Procedural Terminology - Wikipedia. (n.d.). Retrieved October 21, 2016, from https://en.wikipedia.org/wiki/Current_Procedural_Terminology

ICD-10 (ICD is new)

ICD - ICD-10 - International Classification of Diseases ... (n.d.). Retrieved October 21, 2016, from http://www.cdc.gov/nchs/icd/icd10.htm

Provider Numbers (*Some Providers that Have NPI Numbers*)

National Provider Identifier - Wikipedia. (n.d.). Retrieved October 21, 2016, from https://en.wikipedia.org/wiki/National_Provider_Identifier

Place of Service Codes (*Common Place of Service Code List*)

Place of Service Code Set - Centers for Medicare ... (n.d.). Retrieved October 21, 2016, from http://www.cms.gov/Medicare/Coding/place-of-service-codes/Place_of_Service_Code_Set.html

Clearinghouse (*Edits a Clearinghouse Can Check For*)

Information Access Management: Isolating Healthcare ... (n.d.). Retrieved October 21, 2016, from http://www.hipaa.com/information-access-management-isolating-healthcare-clearinghouse-functions-what-to-do-and-how-to-do-it/

Medicare Fee Schedule (Image)

Overview of the Medicare Physician Fee Schedule Search. (n.d.). Retrieved October 21, 2016, from http://www.cms.gov/apps/physician-fee-schedule/overview.aspx

How to Appeal Medicare (Appeal Levels of Medicare)

Medicare Parts A & B Appeals Process - cms.gov. (n.d.). Retrieved October 21, 2016, from http://www.cms.gov/Outreach-and-Education/Medicare-Learning-Network-MLN/MLNProducts/Downloads/MedicareAppealsProcess.pdf

How to Complete a CMS 1500 (CMS 1500 form)

CMS Forms - Centers for Medicare & Medicaid Services. (n.d.). Retrieved October 21, 2016, from http://www.cms.gov/Medicare/CMS-Forms/CMS-Forms/index.html

How to Issue an ABN

Medicare Advance Beneficiary Notices - cms.gov. (n.d.). Retrieved October 21, 2016, from http://www.cms.gov/Outreach-and-Education/Medicare-Learning-Network-MLN/MLNProducts/Downloads/ABN_Booklet_ICN006266.pdf

ABOUT THE AUTHORS

Rochelle and Ashley are a mother/daughter team who decided 2016 was the year to step out on faith. For years, Rochelle has had this dream of using her experience as a way to change the way she currently navigates though life. Ashley, an educator with a new baby at home, wanted the exact same thing.

Knowing Rochelle's vast knowledge in the health insurance industry could serve as a means to educate others while at the same time untying them both from their predictable 8 to 5 routines, Ashley convinced her mom to dig up that dream, bury her fears and finally write this book.

Please visit www.1500pays.com

www.ingramcontent.com/pod-product-compliance
Lightning Source LLC
Chambersburg PA
CBHW080615190526
45169CB00009B/3194